Bowel Imaging

Editor

JORDI RIMOLA

MAGNETIC RESONANCE IMAGING CLINICS OF NORTH AMERICA

www.mri.theclinics.com

Consulting Editors
SURESH K. MUKHERJI
LYNNE S. STEINBACH

February 2014 • Volume 22 • Number 1

ELSEVIER

1600 John F. Kennedy Boulevard • Suite 1800 • Philadelphia, Pennsylvania, 19103-2899

http://www.mri.theclinics.com

MRI CLINICS OF NORTH AMERICA Volume 22, Number 1
February 2014 ISSN 1064-9689, ISBN 13: 978-0-323-26666-6

Editor: John Vassallo (j.vassallo@elsevier.com)
Developmental Editor: Yonah Korngold

Magnetic Resonance Imaging Clinics of North America (ISSN 1064-9689) is published quarterly by Elsevier Inc., 360 Park Avenue South, New York, NY 10010-1710. Months of issue are February, May, August, and November. Business and Editorial Offices: 1600 John F. Kennedy Blvd., Ste. 1800, Philadelphia, PA 19103-2899. Customer Service Office: 3251 Riverport Lane, Maryland Heights, MO 63043. Periodicals postage paid at New York, NY and additional mailing offices. Subscription prices are $375.00 per year (domestic individuals), $581.00 per year (domestic institutions), $190.00 per year (domestic students/residents), $420.00 per year (Canadian individuals), $755.00 per year (Canadian institutions), $545.00 per year (international individuals), $755.00 per year (international institutions), and $275.00 per year (international and Canadian students/residents). International air speed delivery is included in all *Clinics* subscription prices. All prices are subject to change without notice. **POSTMASTER:** Send address changes to *Magnetic Resonance Imaging Clinics*, Elsevier Health Sciences Division, Subscription Customer Service, 3251 Riverport Lane, Maryland Heights, MO 63043. Customer Service (orders, claims, online, change of address): Elsevier Health Sciences Division, Subscription Customer Service, 3251 Riverport Lane, Maryland Heights, MO 63043. Tel:1-800-654-2452 (U.S. and Canada); 314-447-8871 (outside U.S. and Canada). Fax: 314-447-8029. E-mail: journalscustomerservice-usa@elsevier.com (for print support); journalsonlinesupport-usa@elsevier.com (for online support).

Reprints. For copies of 100 or more of articles in this publication, please contact the Commercial Reprints Department, Elsevier Inc., 360 Park Avenue South, New York, NY 10010-1710. Tel.: 212-633-3874; Fax: 212-633-3820; E-mail: reprints@elsevier.com.

Magnetic Resonance Imaging Clinics of North America is covered in the *RSNA Index of Imaging Literature, MEDLINE/PubMed (Index Medicus),* and *EMBASE/Excerpta Medica.*

Printed and bound by CPI Group (UK) Ltd, Croydon, CR0 4YY

Transferred to digital print 2012

Contributors

CONSULTING EDITORS

SURESH K. MUKHERJI, MD, FACR
Professor and Chairman; W.F. Patenge
Endowed Chair, Department of Radiology,
Michigan State University, East Lansing,
Michigan

LYNNE S. STEINBACH, MD, FACR
Professor of Clinical Radiology and
Orthopaedic Surgery, University of
California-San Francisco, San Francisco,
California

EDITOR

JORDI RIMOLA, MD, PhD
Department of Radiology, Hospital Clínic of
Barcelona, CIBER-EHD, IDIBAPS, University of
Barcelona, Barcelona, Spain

AUTHORS

MAHMOUD M. AL-HAWARY, MD
Associate Professor and Section Chief
Gastrointestinal Radiology, Department of
Radiology, University of Michigan Hospitals,
Ann Arbor, Michigan

REGINA G.H. BEETS-TAN, MD, PhD
Department of Radiology, Maastricht
University Medical Center, Maastricht,
The Netherlands

DIDIER BIELEN, MD, PhD
Department of Radiology, University Hospitals
Leuven; Department of Imaging and Pathology,
KU Leuven, Leuven, Belgium

GIANFRANCO GUALDI, MD
Radiology Department, Umberto I Hospital,
Sapienza University, Rome, Italy

VIVEK GOWDRA HALAPPA, MD
Department of Radiology and Radiological
Sciences, The Johns Hopkins University
School of Medicine, Baltimore, Maryland

HERO K. HUSSAIN, MD
Associate Professor and Section Chief Body
MRI, Department of Radiology, University of
Michigan Hospitals, Ann Arbor, Michigan

IHAB KAMEL, MD, PhD
Department of Radiology and Radiological
Sciences, The Johns Hopkins University
School of Medicine, Baltimore, Maryland

FRANCESCA LAGHI, MD
Radiology Department, Umberto I Hospital,
Sapienza University, Rome, Italy

GABRIELE MASSELLI, MD
Radiology Department, Umberto I Hospital,
Sapienza University, Rome, Italy

RICCARDO MONTI, MD
Radiology Department, Umberto I Hospital,
Sapienza University, Rome, Italy

INGRID ORDÁS, MD
Department of Gastroenterology, Hospital
Clínic Barcelona, CIBER-EHD, IDIBAPS,
University of Barcelona, Barcelona, Spain

AYTEKIN OTO, MD
Department of Radiology, University of
Chicago, Chicago, Illinois

ELISABETTA POLETTINI, MD
Radiology Department, Umberto I Hospital,
Sapienza University, Rome, Italy

JORDI RIMOLA, MD, PhD
Department of Radiology, Hospital Clínic of
Barcelona, CIBER-EHD, IDIBAPS, University of
Barcelona, Barcelona, Spain

CYNTHIA S. SANTILLAN, MD
Chief of Computed Tomography; Vice-Chief of
Body Imaging Section; Associate Professor of
Radiology, Department of Radiology,
University of California San Diego, San Diego,
California

JAAP STOKER, MD, PhD
Department of Radiology, Academic Medical
Center, University of Amsterdam, Amsterdam,
The Netherlands

MICHAEL R. TORKZAD, MD, PhD
Section of Radiology, Department of
Radiology, Oncology and Radiation Science,
Uppsala University, Uppsala, Sweden

GERT VAN ASSCHE, MD, PhD
Department of Gastroenterology, University
Hospitals Leuven; Department of Clinical and
Experimental Medicine, KU Leuven, Leuven,
Belgium

DIRK VANBECKEVOORT, MD
Department of Radiology, University Hospitals
Leuven, Leuven, Belgium

MARIJE P. VAN DER PAARDT, MD
Department of Radiology, Academic Medical
Center, University of Amsterdam, Amsterdam,
The Netherlands

RAGNA VANSLEMBROUCK, MD
Department of Radiology, University Hospitals
Leuven, Leuven, Belgium

JOSEPH H. YACOUB, MD
Department of Radiology, Northwestern
University, Chicago, Illinois

ELLEN M. ZIMMERMANN, MD
Professor, Department of Internal
Medicine/Gastroenterology, University of
Michigan Hospitals, Ann Arbor, Michigan

Contents

> Due to advances in technology, magnetic resonance is an increasingly popular method for evaluating the small bowel and colon because of the lack of radiation, wealth of information provided by the images, and growing demand from gastroenterologists, surgeons, and oncologists. Careful attention to proper technique, however, is necessary to obtain high-quality images. Factors that need to be considered for successful magnetic resonance of the bowel include the method for administration of oral or rectal contrast, patient positioning, the need for antiperistaltic medication, and imaging sequences and planes.

> MR enterography has an established role in evaluating patients with Crohn disease, providing essential complementary information to clinical assessment, and as an indispensible adjunct to clinical tools such as colonoscopy. MR enterography examinations can establish the diagnosis of Crohn disease, evaluate disease activity and complications, and assess treatment response, thus providing support for clinical decision-making. Currently, MR imaging findings are highly predictive of tissue inflammation and can be used clinically to guide clinical care.

> MR colonography has a high diagnostic accuracy for detecting Crohn disease (CD) activity and determining the extent and severity of lesions. In the setting of stricturing CD, MR colonography can provide a detailed map of the lesions, which is useful for clinical decision making. MR colonography can be used as an alternative to conventional colonoscopy in the setting of CD, or as a complementary tool in selected patients with ulcerative colitis. This article reviews the spectrum of MR colonography findings in colonic inflammatory bowel disease and discusses the potential applications and limitations of MR colonography.

> Magnetic resonance (MR) enterography has an increasing role in the evaluation of the small bowel in patients with Crohn disease. MR enterography is accurate for

disease assessment and can influence the choice of therapy. Functional sequences may increase the role of MR enterography in Crohn disease. Techniques such as high-resolution MR enterography, diffusion-weighted imaging, dynamic contrast-enhanced MR imaging, magnetization transfer, and MR motility imaging may allow better assessment of disease extent, activity, and severity. Quantitative analysis using these advanced techniques as well as the standard techniques may provide methods for evaluating and following the disease in the future.

Magnetic resonance (MR) imaging has been playing an evolving role in evaluating noninflammatory small-bowel conditions, such as tumors and malabsorption syndrome. MR imaging has shown to be superior to other diagnostic methods in identifying tumors of the small bowel. MR enterography and MR enteroclysis are both valid for studying noninflammatory conditions of the small intestine, although MR enteroclysis may be considered the modality of choice because of its accuracy in the diagnosis of small-bowel neoplasms. Intraluminal and extraluminal MR findings, combined with contrast-agent enhancement and functional information, help to make an accurate diagnosis and consequently to characterize small-bowel diseases.

Colorectal cancer is the second most common cause of cancer-related death in Europe and the United States, and a major cause of mortality. Early detection of colorectal cancer and its precursors reduces mortality and morbidity, and a minimally invasive screening tool is essential for high patient acceptance and participation. To achieve this goal, computed tomographic colonography and magnetic resonance (MR) colonography have been introduced. A wide variety of methods of bowel preparation, colon distension, and imaging exists for MR colonography. This article presents an up-to-date overview of the status of MR colonography in screening for colorectal cancer, and its diagnosis.

Magnetic resonance imaging plays a pivotal role in the imaging and staging of rectal and anal carcinomas. Rectal adenocarcinomas and anal squamous cell carcinomas behave differently, and are staged and treated differently. This article attempts to explain these 2 entities, which share the same regions of interest, in a comprehensive manner.

Perianal fistulization is the result of a chronic inflammation of the perianal tissues. A wide spectrum of clinical manifestations, ranging from simple to complex fistulas, can be seen, the latter especially in patients with Crohn disease. Failure to detect secondary tracks and hidden abscesses may lead to therapeutic failure, such as insufficient response to medical treatment and relapse after surgery. Currently, magnetic resonance (MR) imaging is the preferred technique for evaluating perianal fistulas and associated complications. Initially used most often in the preoperative setting, MR imaging now also plays an important role in evaluating the response to medical therapy.

MAGNETIC RESONANCE IMAGING CLINICS OF NORTH AMERICA

RELATED INTEREST

Neuroimaging Clinics, **August 2013**
MR Spectroscopy of the Brain
Lara A. Brandão, *Editor*

DOWNLOAD Free App!

Review Articles
THE CLINICS

NOW AVAILABLE FOR YOUR iPhone and iPad

PROGRAM OBJECTIVE
The goal of Magnetic Resonance Imaging Clinics of North America is to keep practicing physicians up to date with current clinical practice by providing timely articles reviewing the state of the art in patient care.

TARGET AUDIENCE
All practicing physicians and healthcare professionals who provide patient care utilizing findings from Magnetic Resonance Imaging.

LEARNING OBJECTIVES
Upon completion of this activity, participants will be able to:
1. Recognize MR imaging of the small bowel in Crohn's Disease, rectal and anal cancer, and perianal fistulas.
2. Review Non inflammatory conditions of the small bowel.
3. Discuss MR colonography in inflammatory bowel disease and the screening and diagnosis of colorectal cancer.

ACCREDITATION
The Elsevier Office of Continuing Medical Education (EOCME) is accredited by the Accreditation Council for Continuing Medical Education (ACCME) to provide continuing medical education for physicians.

The EOCME designates this enduring material for a maximum of 15 *AMA PRA Category 1 Credit*(s)™. Physicians should claim only the credit commensurate with the extent of their participation in the activity.

All other health care professionals requesting continuing education credit for this enduring material will be issued a certificate of participation.

DISCLOSURE OF CONFLICTS OF INTEREST
The EOCME assesses conflict of interest with its instructors, faculty, planners, and other individuals who are in a position to control the content of CME activities. All relevant conflicts of interest that are identified are thoroughly vetted by EOCME for fair balance, scientific objectivity, and patient care recommendations. EOCME is committed to providing its learners with CME activities that promote improvements or quality in healthcare and not a specific proprietary business or a commercial interest.

The planning committee, staff, authors and editors listed below have identified no financial relationships or relationships to products or devices they or their spouse/life partner have with commercial interest related to the content of this CME activity:

Mahmoud M. Al-Hawary, MD; Regina G.H. Beets-Tan, MD, PhD; Didier Bielen, MD, PhD; Gianfranco Gualdi, MD; Vivek Gowdra Halappa, MD; Kristen Helm; Brynne Hunter; Hero K. Hussain, MD; Ihab Kamel, MD, PhD; Francesca Laghi, MD; Sandy Lavery; Jill McNair; Gabriele Masselli, MD; Riccardo Monti, MD; Suresh K. Mukherji, MD; Ingrid Ordás, MD; Aytekin Oto, MD; Elisabetta Polettini, MD; Jordi Rimola, MD, PhD; Lynne S. Steinbach, MD, FACR; Jaap Stoker, MD, PhD; Karthikeyan Subramaniam; Michael R. Torkzad, MD, PhD; John Vassallo; Gert Van Assche, MD, PhD; Dirk Vanbeckevoort, MD; Marije P. van der Paardt, MD; Ragna Vanslembrouck, MD; Joseph H. Yacoub, MD; Ellen M. Zimmermann, MD.

The planning committee, staff, authors and editors listed below have identified financial relationships or relationships to products or devices they or their spouse/life partner have with commercial interest related to the content of this CME activity:

Cynthia S. Santillan, MD is a consultant/advisor for Robarts Clinical Research.

UNAPPROVED/OFF-LABEL USE DISCLOSURE
The EOCME requires CME faculty to disclose to the participants:
1. When products or procedures being discussed are off-label, unlabelled, experimental, and/or investigational (not US Food and Drug Administration (FDA) approved); and
2. Any limitations on the information presented, such as data that are preliminary or that represent ongoing research, interim analyses, and/or unsupported opinions. Faculty may discuss information about pharmaceutical agents that is outside of FDA-approved labelling. This information is intended solely for CME and is not intended to promote off-label use of these medications. If you have any questions, contact the medical affairs department of the manufacturer for the most recent prescribing information.

TO ENROLL
To enroll in the *Magnetic Resonance Imaging Clinics of North* Continuing Medical Education program, call customer service at 1-800-654-2452 or sign up online at http://www.theclinics.com/home/cme. The CME program is available to subscribers for an additional annual fee of $223 USD.

METHOD OF PARTICIPATION
In order to claim credit, participants must complete the following:
1. Complete enrolment as indicated above.
2. Read the activity.
3. Complete the CME Test and Evaluation. Participants must achieve a score of 70% on the test. All CME Tests and Evaluations must be completed online.

CME INQUIRIES/SPECIAL NEEDS
For all CME inquiries or special needs, please contact elsevierCME@elsevier.com.

Foreword
Bowel Imaging

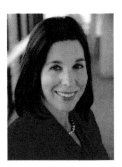

Lynne S. Steinbach, MD, FACR
Consulting Editor

Suresh Mukherji and I are pleased to present this latest issue of *Magnetic Resonance Imaging Clinics of North America* that covers the topic of bowel MR imaging. The guest editor, Jordi Rimola, MD, PhD, is a well-respected abdominal imager from the Hospital Clinic Barcelona in Spain. In addition to himself, he has assembled an impressive cadre of authors from prestigious American and European institutions. These luminaries include Mahmoud Al-Hawary from University of Michigan, Cynthia Santillan from UC San Diego, Joseph Yacoub and Ayetkin Oto from Northwestern University in Chicago, Gabriele Masselli from Umberto I Hospital in Rome, Japp Stoker from the University of Amsterdam in the Netherlands, Michael Torkzad from Uppsala University in Sweden, and Dirk Vanbeckevoort from University of Leuven in Belgium. The topics are timely and the material is cutting edge. With increasing use of MR imaging for bowel imaging made possible by improvements in hardware and software, and the lack of ionizing radiation compared to CT, this compendium of information could not have come out at a better time. We thank all of the authors for their excellent contributions.

Lynne S. Steinbach, MD, FACR
Clinical Radiology and Orthopaedic Surgery
University of California-San Francisco
505 Parnassus
San Francisco, CA 94143-0628, USA

E-mail address:
lynne.steinbach@ucsf.edu

Magn Reson Imaging Clin N Am 22 (2014) xi
http://dx.doi.org/10.1016/j.mric.2013.09.003
1064-9689/14/$ – see front matter © 2014 Published by Elsevier Inc.

Preface
Bowel Imaging

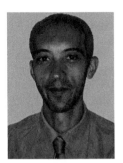

Jordi Rimola, MD, PhD
Editor

This issue of the *Magnetic Resonance Imaging Clinics of North America* is dedicated to imaging of the bowel. Of the eight articles in total, two are focused on technical aspects, both the classic and the new modalities that may potentially improve the accuracy of the technique. Four articles review the role of MR in detecting the inflammatory and noninflammatory conditions of the small and large bowel. Finally, one article focuses on the role of MR in imaging and staging of rectal and anal carcinomas, and the last one discusses the role of MR imaging in the assessment of the fistula in the ano.

The evaluation of the small bowel using conventional endoscopy and radiology is challenging due to its length and caliper. Over the past several years, the use of cross-sectional imaging techniques for suspected small-bowel disorders has increased. Cross-sectional techniques allow visualization of the entire bowel and detection of extraluminal pathologic conditions. Given the fact that most groups of pathologies in the bowel have transmural involvement and cannot be evaluated by endoscopy, this represented another key factor in understanding the implementation of the technique in clinical practice. Due to the increasing awareness of radiation exposure, there has been a more global interest in implementing MR imaging that either reduce or eliminate radiation exposure. This is especially important in patients with chronic diseases such as inflammatory bowel disease, who may require multiple studies over a lifetime, or in studies that require sequential imaging time points such as the assessment of gastrointestinal motility. Besides this, MR imaging has many properties that make it well suited to imaging of the bowel, especially the improved tissue contrast. The intra- and extraluminal MR findings, combined with T2-weighted, contrast enhancement and functional information, help make an accurate diagnosis and consequently characterize bowel diseases.

As with the small bowel, MR imaging evaluation of the colon and the rectum has also undergone significant advances over the past decade. The one-stop shop concept has led to the evaluation of the colon together with the small bowel in the assessment of IBD, thus avoiding the need for colonoscopies in a select group of patients. MR colonography has also emerged as an alternative tool to colonoscopy for both the screening and the diagnosis of colorectal cancer. The use of MR imaging for rectal cancer staging has evolved rapidly in recent years and currently represents part of the standard of care. Finally, the current status of MR imaging in the diagnosis and classification of perianal fistula representing critical data for obtaining a surgical map and the role of MR imaging in fistula follow-up after medical treatment are also reviewed.

Magn Reson Imaging Clin N Am 22 (2014) xiii–xiv
http://dx.doi.org/10.1016/j.mric.2013.09.002

As guest editor of this issue of *Magnetic Resonance Imaging Clinics of North America*, I was fortunate enough to enlist contributions from a number of distinguished abdominal and gastrointestinal radiologists, as well as from younger investigators with experience in the field of bowel imagery. My intention was to cover all aspects of MR imaging of the bowel in detail. Some overlap was inescapable, although it perhaps provides differing points of view. I express my gratitude to all the authors for their generous contributions in sharing their cutting-edge knowledge and expertise in the different topics. I am sure that this issue will become a valuable tool for radiologists as well as clinicians who are aware of the impact of MR imaging on their management of patients.

Jordi Rimola, MD, PhD
Department of Radiology
Hospital Clínic of Barcelona
University of Barcelona
Villarroel 170, Barcelona, 08036 Catalonia, Spain

E-mail address:
jrimola@clinic.ub.es

MR Imaging Techniques of the Bowel

Cynthia S. Santillan, MD

KEYWORDS

- Small bowel • Colon • Magnetic resonance enterography • Magnetic resonance colonography
- Inflammatory bowel disease • Crohn disease

KEY POINTS

- Magnetic resonance (MR) enterography is imaging of the small bowel following administration of a large volume of oral contrast and is now a recommended method of imaging for patients with inflammatory bowel disease, particularly in young patients.
- MR colonography is imaging of the colon following administration of air or fluid via the rectum after the patient has completed a bowel cleansing preparation or fecal tagging.
- Antiperistaltic medications are recommended for both MR enterography and colonography to decrease blurring and prevent bowel spasm that may mimic pathologic abnormality.
- Rapid imaging sequences are necessary to delineate anatomy, detect polyps or masses, and evaluate bowel wall thickness and signal characteristics.

INTRODUCTION

Cross-sectional imaging has become an important and increasingly used method for the assessment of the small bowel and colon.[1,2] Magnetic resonance (MR) and computed tomographic (CT) imaging can provide information not available endoscopically such as transmural pathologic abnormality and disease in the adjacent tissues and organs. Also, MR and CT enterography and colonography are less invasive than endoscopy and do not have the risks of obstruction and device retention that are associated with capsule endoscopy. Current guidelines recommend CT and MR enterography as the imaging techniques of choice for assessing patients with Crohn disease.[3]

Although CT imaging of the bowel has been preferred in the past over MR because of bowel motion, artifacts, and limits on spatial resolution and coverage, recent advances in MR technology have made it possible to generate high-quality images of the entire bowel, allowing assessment of anatomy, fold patterns, wall thickness, masses, and inflammation. MR enterography and colonography offer several advantages over their CT counterparts. MR imaging is a radiation-free alternative to CT imaging, which is an important feature, given current concerns about radiation exposure from medical imaging.[4] Cumulative radiation is a particular concern in young patients with inflammatory bowel disease who will require a lifetime of imaging as well as for patients who require screening for small bowel (such as Peutz Jeger) or colonic neoplasms.[5] Because of its lack of radiation, multiple postcontrast phases can be performed with little additional risk to the patient, which can allow better characterization of pathologic abnormality. In addition, imaging at multiple time points along with cine imaging can facilitate distinction between peristalsis and stenosis in the bowel and can provide functional information on motility. MR imaging can also provide information that cannot be assessed on CT imaging, such as diffusivity.

Disclosure – Consultant, Robarts Clinical Research.
Department of Radiology, University of California San Diego, 200 West Arbor Drive #8756, San Diego, CA 92120, USA
E-mail address: csantillan@ucsd.edu

Magn Reson Imaging Clin N Am 22 (2014) 1–11
http://dx.doi.org/10.1016/j.mric.2013.07.004
1064-9689/14/$ – see front matter © 2014 Elsevier Inc. All rights reserved.

The following article presents guidelines for the performance of MR enterography and colonography, including discussions of options for bowel distension, imaging sequences, and need for patient preparation or medication.

EQUIPMENT

To achieve adequate spatial resolution, MR enterography should be performed on a system capable of a field strength of 1.5 T or greater. Increasing availability of 3-T systems will likely result in more MR enterography studies performed at higher field strengths. When transitioning to a 3-T protocol, however, some sequences may need to be modified, particularly T2-weighted imaging, to address increased artifacts and higher specific absorption rates.[6,7] A phased array coil or combination of phased array coils that can provide coverage of the entire abdomen and pelvis is necessary to image the entire bowel in the coronal plane.

PATIENT SCREENING

As with other MR techniques, patients should be screened for contraindications to MR imaging or factors that may compromise image quality or the patient's ability to complete the examination. Patients should be screened for the presence of pacemakers, other devices, or foreign bodies that may malfunction or move due to the scanner's magnetic field or imaging sequences.[8] Surgical clips in the abdomen and pelvis can result in extensive artifacts based on their composition. Prior MR and CT examinations and their reports should be reviewed for evidence of significant artifact so a decision can be made at the time of scheduling or protocolling as to whether CT or MR imaging is likely to provide the best quality examination for the indication. Artifact related to hip prostheses can pose a particular problem for assessment of the rectum and perianal region. In those patients that MR is preferred or necessary compared with CT, imaging sequences may need to be modified to provide the best information possible.

Claustrophobic or anxious patients need to be reassured that they will have a constant ability to notify the technologist if they need to pause or terminate the examination. Anxiolytics and sedatives should be prescribed with caution, as they may compromise the patient's ability to comply with breathing instructions.

For examinations that will require intravenous gadolinium contrast, patients should be screened for renal insufficiency or prior allergic reactions to contrast.[9]

PATIENT PREPARATION

Patient preparation is determined by the need for colonic filling and bowel cleansing. For a small bowel examination, patients are asked to abstain from solid foods for 6 hours before the examination to reduce particulate material in the bowel during the study. Otherwise, patients do not require any additional preparation or dietary restriction for small bowel imaging.

If colonic imaging is desired, patients may be asked to undergo a bowel cleansing preparation similar to that used for colonoscopy, which usually requires the ingestion of a large volume of polyethylene glycol solution beginning the day before the examination. Many patients state the bowel cleanse is the most uncomfortable part of colonic examinations.[10] To increase patient acceptance of colonography, investigators are exploring fecal tagging with agents demonstrating low signal on T1-weighted imaging such as barium or iron.[11] As part of the preparation with fecal tagging, patients may need to avoid fiber-rich foods and foods that contain manganese, such as chocolate, fruits, and nuts, for 2 days before the examination. Manganese appears bright on T1-weighted imaging, which can interfere with the interpretation of the contrast-enhanced images. Current tagging techniques, however, may not perform well enough for widespread clinical use and patient experience with the technique is mixed.[12,13]

SMALL BOWEL CONTRAST

Appropriate selection and administration of oral contrast is critical to achieve adequate and uniform distension of the small bowel. Oral contrast agents can be described as positive (high signal on both T1- and T2-weighted imaging), negative (low on both T1 and T2), or biphasic. Although many agents have been used for MR enterography, biphasic agents are most widely used.[14–16] The currently preferred agents are low signal on T1-weighted imaging, because high intraluminal signal can obscure abnormal mural enhancement following intravenous contrast administration.[14] Although low intraluminal signal on T2-weighted imaging can improve detection of bowel wall edema, extraluminal fluid, and abscesses, negative contrast agents are more expensive and are not as well tolerated by patients.[14–16]

Water is a well-tolerated and inexpensive biphasic oral contrast; however, rapid absorption by the small bowel often results in poor distension of the distal ileum.[17–19] Several biphasic agents containing osmotic (including mannitol, sorbitol, polyethylene glycol) or bulk-forming (methylcellulose, psyllium) additives are currently available. Some studies suggest that osmotic agents may provide better distension than bulk-forming agents.[17,18] At the author's institution, they use a low concentration (0.1%) barium sulfate suspension containing sorbitol (VoLumen; E-Z-EM, Westbury, NY) for both CT and MR enterography. Apart from mild diarrhea and cramping experienced by some patients, biphasic agents are typically well-tolerated. Because of the large volume ingested, patients are encouraged to urinate before entering the scanner.

Administration of oral contrast requires both sufficient volume and appropriate timing to achieve uniform distension of the bowel (**Fig. 1**). Most protocols require 1.5 L to 2 L of oral contrast administered over the course of 40 to 60 minutes.[20] At the author's institution, the patient is given 450 mL of contrast every 20 minutes beginning 1 hour before the examination for a total of 3 doses. Approximately 450 mL water is given just before entering the magnet. Because the final dose is only for distension of the proximal small bowel and duodenum, hyperosmolar contrast is not necessary. Pediatric patients may receive a smaller dose, typically based on weight.[21,22]

Although most outpatients can complete the oral contrast protocol, some patients cannot or will not ingest the full dose of contrast. It is encouraged that both the ordering physicians and the radiologist discuss the importance of oral contrast with their patients. For those patients that are unable to complete the entire oral contrast protocol, the examination is performed using the contrast they have been able to drink and will include any limitation of the examination due to inadequate distension in the report. Patients that are acutely ill, particularly inpatients, are screened and often

a different examination is recommended in patients who are currently vomiting or are otherwise unable to drink contrast due to pain or altered mental status. If a patient seems to be ill due to an obstruction, however, the procedure will often proceed despite the patient being unable to drink, if a discussion with the referring clinician indicates that acuity of inflammation at the point of obstruction is critical for patient management. As there is often sufficient fluid in the bowel to distend the bowel upstream to the obstruction, oral contrast may not be necessary in these cases. For patients with an acute obstruction, however, the radiologist should contact the ordering physician to see if a CT can provide the necessary information without performing the longer MR enterography.

MR enteroclysis uses an alternative method for bowel distension. MR enteroclysis requires placement of a nasojejunal tube under fluoroscopy, usually an 8-Fr tube because larger tubes are associated with more patient discomfort and may require sedation for the procedure.[23] After confirming the position of the tube distal to the ligament of Treitz, 1 to 2 L of oral contrast is administered manually or with an automated pump. Filling is monitored with intermittent coronal fluid–sensitive imaging to confirm distension of the bowel to the cecum, at which point the infusion is stopped and the MR examination is performed. The decision to perform MR enteroclysis rather than MR enterography is based on several factors, including radiologist experience, indication for the examination, and time available for the examination including tube placement. Currently, MR enteroclysis is performed at fewer institutions than are MR enterography. At centers that perform both examinations, MR enteroclysis is the preferred examination for most small bowel imaging, and MR

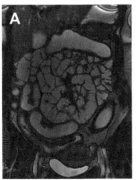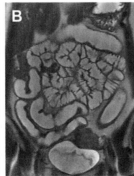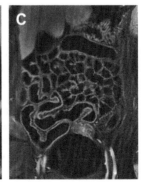

Fig. 1. Coronal bSSFP (A), SSFSE (B), and T1-weighted fat-saturated postcontrast (C) images demonstrate excellent distension of the entire small bowel and portions of the transverse and descending colon. Note the normal fold pattern present in the jejunum and decreased folds in the diseased ileum in the right lower quadrant. The visible portions of the transverse and descending colon also demonstrate decreased haustration. Note increasing bladder distension during the examination due to the large volume of ingested fluid.

enterography is reserved for follow-up in patients with known Crohn disease.[23,24]

COLONIC CONTRAST

Agents for distension of the colon are characterized as either dark-lumen or bright-lumen agents based on their appearance on T1-weighted imaging. Bright-lumen techniques require the rectal administration of fluid containing a dilute gadolinium chelate.[25] The primary imaging sequence for bright-lumen colonography is a 3D T1-weighted fat-saturated sequence whereby masses are visible as filling defects. Intravenous contrast is usually not necessary for bright-lumen colonography, as the bright-lumen content limits assessment of enhancement of the wall and any masses. Because the distinction between stool, air, and masses can be difficult with bright-lumen agents, many institutions prefer dark-lumen agents.[25–27]

Dark-lumen colonography can be performed with either air or water. Air insufflation can be performed with room air or carbon dioxide. Carbon dioxide can be instilled using an automated device similar to what is currently used for CT colonography. The automatic insufflator should remain active during the examination to maintain consistent pressure, as ongoing absorption of carbon dioxide by the colon during the examination may lead to alterations in distension.[28] An advantage of air over fluid for colonic filling is the decreased risk of fecal spillage.

Fluid distension of the colon requires administration of up 2.5 L of warm tap water per rectum, although 1 L may be sufficient in some patients. The fluid is allowed to flow via gravity from a bag positioned about 1 m above the patient, and filling is stopped when either all of the water has been given or the patient begins to feel increasing pressure or discomfort. When performed in conjunction with an MR enterography, the volume tolerated by the patient may be lower because of partial antegrade filling from oral contrast. The rectal tube remains in place until the conclusion of the examination, at which point the fluid can be allowed to drain by gravity back into the bag by placing it on the floor. There is currently conflicting evidence regarding the performance of air versus water for dark-lumen colonography. Although air could result in artifacts on MR imaging, Ajaj and colleagues[29] found no statistical difference in image quality between the 2 methods and contrast-to-noise was thought to be superior on the air examination. In a more recent publication, however, Rodriguez Gomez and colleagues[30] found significantly better distension and less

artifacts in subjects with water compared with air distension. The degree of distension during filling for either method can be monitored using intermittent coronal imaging with either gradient echo (for bright lumen) or rapid fluid sensitive sequences (for dark lumen).

Oral contrast has been explored as an alternative to per rectal distension of the colon. The method requires the ingestion of 2 to 2.5 L of contrast, a larger volume than used for small bowel imaging, over the course of 1 to 2 hours before the examination. This method was shown to achieve adequate colonic distension by Bakir and colleagues[31] and may be an alternative method for colonic filling in select patients.

POSITIONING

The author performs MR of the small bowel with the patient in the prone position when possible because it offers several advantages to supine positioning. Positioning the patient prone decreases the anterior-posterior diameter of the abdomen, allowing for better spatial resolution for any given imaging time when acquiring images in the coronal plane (**Fig. 2**). Bowel distension is improved in the prone position.[32] Prone positioning also results in compression of the abdomen, allowing separation of the bowel loops. For patients that cannot tolerate the prone position, because of an ostomy or other source of discomfort, the examination can be performed in the supine position.

For patients undergoing bright-lumen MR colonography, the examination requires imaging in both the supine and the prone position to displace colonic air and fecal material. If a dark-lumen agent is used, particularly in combination with fecal tagging, imaging may be performed in either position or both based on institutional preference.[25]

COVERAGE

Coronal sequences and coil positioning should be optimized to include the entire small bowel and colon. The coronal plane allows for visualization of the maximum amount of bowel on a single image, which aids in detection of bowel that is abnormally thickened, hyperenhancing, or isolated from other loops of bowel due to fibrofatty proliferation of the mesentery. Although dedicated views of the rectum and perianal region are discussed in a separate article, routine MR enterography studies should attempt to include this region in at least one series. To achieve adequate coverage of the pelvis, portions of the spleen and liver may need to be excluded, which is considered appropriate in this setting.[33] When starting a bowel MR

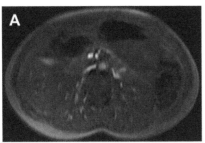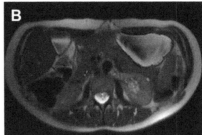

Fig. 2. Localizer image in the supine position (A) compared with an SSFSE image in the prone position (B) of the same patient demonstrates the difference in the anteroposterior diameter of the abdomen between the 2 positions. The shorter distance that needs to be covered in the prone position during coronal imaging allows for either increased spatial resolution or shorter breath-holds, particularly during 3D gradient echo postcontrast imaging.

program, radiologists should work closely with their technologists, because they may not be accustomed to extending anterior and caudal coverage on the coronal images to include the entire bowel.

ANTI-PERISTALTICS

Anti-peristaltic agents are routinely administered at many institutions to decrease bowel motion, particularly during the contrast-enhanced dynamic imaging, because the 3D acquisition is very sensitive to motion. Although many of the sequences for MR enterography are relatively rapid, the benefits of reduced flow artifacts on the single-shot fast spin-echo (SSFSE) sequences and decreased blurring likely outweigh the relatively low risk of adverse effects associated with the medication.

Glucagon, which is the antiperistaltic available in the United States, or hyoscine N-butylbromide should be given to all patients undergoing MR enterography or colonography unless it is contraindicated due to diabetes or pregnancy. Most protocols involve the administration of 0.5 mg to 1 mg glucagon or 20 mg to 40 mg hyoscine. The intravenous route for either agent provides effect within 85 seconds compared with at least 5 minutes for an intramuscular injection.[34,35] Duration of spasmolysis has been shown to be approximately 20 minutes for both agents, although Froehlich and colleagues[34] reported that hyoscine had a significantly shorter duration at 7 minutes.[35] Intramuscular administration of either agent results in a delay of onset of spasmolysis, at least 5 minutes, without a significant change in the duration of spasmolysis compared with intravenous administration.[35] Depending on the length of the examination, the medication can be administered as a split dose rather than a single administration to provide more consistent spasmolysis for the duration of the examination. In patients who are undergoing

colonic distension, the first dose should be given at the time of filling to minimize colonic spasm. Intravenous injection of anti-peristaltic medications should be performed slowly to avoid nausea or vomiting. For small bowel imaging at the author's institution, they administer the first slow intravenous injection of 0.5 mg glucagon after performing cine imaging at the beginning of the examination, and the second 0.5 mg IV dose just before contrast administration.

INTRAVENOUS CONTRAST AND POSTCONTRAST IMAGING

Contrast-enhanced imaging is an important part of the MR enterography examination and all examinations should be performed with contrast unless there is a contraindication to gadolinium intravenous contrast. In patients at risk for nephrogenic systemic fibrosis due to severe renal insufficiency, pregnant patients, or patients with an allergy to gadolinium contrast, the MR enterography can be performed without contrast. If the patient is on hemodialysis, CT enterography with iodinated contrast is a reasonable alternative. For MR colonography, dark-lumen colonography should always be performed with intravenous contrast; however, intravenous contrast may not be necessary for bright-lumen colonography as previously discussed. Patients are given a standard dose of 0.1 mmol/kg gadolinium contrast at 2 mL per second followed by a saline flush. The images are obtained with a 3D fat-saturated gradient echo sequence in the coronal plane to minimize imaging time while covering the entire bowel. The author has found that many young patients can comfortably tolerate a breath-hold of up to 25 seconds, which allows for thin slices of 3 mm or less. The technologists are then asked to make allowances in larger patients or if the patient cannot hold his breath long enough to obtain adequate coverage, but to not exceed a slice thickness of 3.5 mm.

The timing of the postcontrast imaging varies at different institutions. Peak small bowel enhancement has varied on multiple studies, ranging from 49 to 85 seconds after contrast.[36–38] Peak enhancement of inflamed segments on MR enterography, however, may occur earlier at 20 to 40 seconds after contrast.[38,39] Despite this difference, it is not clear whether imaging closer to 40 seconds than 70 seconds provides an improved ability to identify and characterize diseased segments.[40] At the author's institution, they begin obtaining the first postcontrast phase 20 seconds after contrast injection and the typical sequence length is 20 to 25 seconds. They obtain 2 additional phases at approximately 90 seconds and 3 minutes after contrast injection. They find obtaining multiple early phases useful because they are often able to obtain at least one early phase free of respiratory motion artifact in most patients. In patients being assessed for a small bowel neoplasm, multiple phases may aid in identification of a mass because of different enhancement characteristics between the mass and adjacent bowel. An axial 2D fat-suppressed T1-weighted series may also be performed following contrast administration, which can aid in localization of extraintestinal findings and delineation of fistulas and sinus tracts.

RAPID FLUID-SENSITIVE SEQUENCES

Rapid fluid-sensitive imaging is critical for assessment of bowel anatomy and inflammation. Although MR colonography performed for inflammatory bowel disease should include fluid-sensitive sequences, screening for polyps and masses with dark-lumen techniques may be performed using only T1-weighted imaging.[41] The 2 most commonly used fluid-sensitive sequences, balanced steady-state free-precession (bSSFP) and SSFSE, are typically used in a combination of axial and coronal planes due to their different strengths and weaknesses.

bSSFP sequences are extremely fast, resulting in crisp images without motion artifact. Their clarity and high signal-to-noise ratio (SNR) allow for good visualization of bowel folds and anatomy, which can sometimes be a challenge in patients with multiple prior surgeries. Kinking and tethering of loops that can suggest fistulas and sinus tracts are also well demonstrated on this sequence. bSSFP images also provide an excellent assessment of the bowel lumen, as they do not have the flow artifacts that can complicate SSFSE imaging. As the bSSFP sequence is often acquired at a time to echo at or near out-of-phase, chemical shift artifact aids characterization of vessels and identification of lymph nodes and edema within the mesenteric fat. Chemical shift artifact can also demonstrate submucosal fat within the bowel wall. Limitations of bSSFP sequences include greater sensitivity to susceptibility artifacts from intraluminal gas and surgical material than seen with SSFSE imaging (**Fig. 3**). As the contrast of bSSFP sequences represents the ratio between T2 and T1, the resulting signal from the bowel wall and solid viscera can be relatively homogeneous and bland, making the sequence insensitive for the presence of edema or solid lesions within these structures (**Fig. 4**).[42,43]

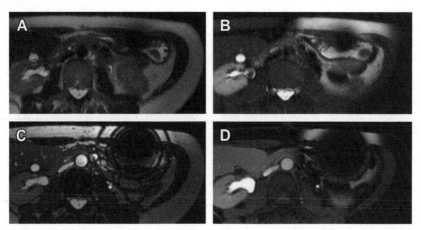

Fig. 3. Axial SSFSE image demonstrates loss of signal in the right lower quadrant due to a surgical clip (*A*). Note how the axial SSFSE image with fat saturation (*B*) demonstrates that the area of field disruption is larger than the region of loss of signal on the image without fat saturation. Susceptibility artifact markedly limits assessment of the right lower quadrant on both the bSSFP (*C*) and the gradient recalled T1-weighted images (*D*).

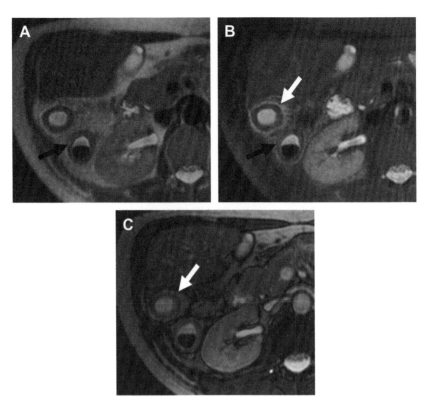

Fig. 4. Axial SSFSE (*A*), fat-saturated SSFSE (*B*) and bSSFP (*C*) images demonstrate thickening of the hepatic flexure of the colon. Mural edema is best appreciated on the SSFSE images, particularly with fat saturation (*black arrows*). The surrounding mesenteric edema is best seen on the bSSFP and fat-saturated SSFSE images (*white arrows*).

SSFSE sequences are also very fast, enabling assessment of small bowel anatomy and wall thickness. As opposed to bSSFP, SSFSE sequences are more purely T2-weighted, allowing for better assessment of bowel wall edema and free fluid. Variable success has been found with more heavily T2-weighted sequences, such as fast spin-echo, due to motion artifact that can render the images uninterpretable above the low pelvis or perirectal region. After reviewing the images and history, sagittal SSFSE imaging may also be performed for assessment of complex fistulas and sinus tracts above the pelvis, particularly those that extend to the anterior abdominal wall. Limitations of SSFSE imaging include greater sensitivity to motion and a lower SNR compared with bSSFP. SSFSE sequences should be performed following the administration of anti-peristaltic medication to minimize blurring and intraluminal flow artifacts from peristalsis (**Fig. 5**). The author typically performs bSSFP sequences first in the protocol, to make sure the anti-peristaltic has taken effect before performing the SSFSE sequences.

Fat-saturated fluid-sensitive images can aid detection of mural and mesenteric edema. Identification of edema is necessary for both interpretation of the images and scoring of disease activity in several of the indices currently under development.[44] Fat saturation also aids assessment of the patency of fistulas and sinus tracts. There is no consensus on whether bSSFP or SSFSE is preferable for fat-saturated imaging.[24] At the author's institution, they use fat saturation on an axial SSFSE sequence. In patients with metallic clips or hip prostheses that result in field inhomogeneities, short inversion time inversion recovery sequences can be used for more reliable fat suppression than chemical fat suppression. Short inversion time inversion recovery sequences can take longer to perform, however, and are typically best suited for relatively immobile portions of the pelvis, such as the rectum and perianal region.

Fluid-sensitive sequences should be performed with a combination of coronal and axial planes. Slice thickness should be 4 to 5 mm to facilitate assessment of anatomy and detect small abnormalities, such as ulcers or fistulas. Images should

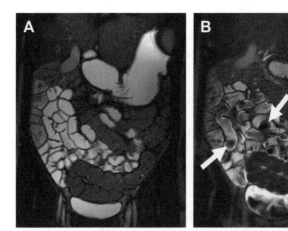

Fig. 5. Coronal bSSFP image demonstrates homogeneous bright signal within the lumen of the small bowel (*A*). Coronal SSFSE image demonstrates multiple foci of low signal in the bowel representing intraluminal flow artifacts, which can limit assessment of luminal or mucosal masses (*arrows, B*).

be performed without interleaving different breath-holds if possible, because variability in the patient's breaths can make it difficult to follow the bowel. Ultimately, the decision of which fluid-sensitive sequences to perform and in which planes should be based on a combination of the information provided by each sequence and the relative quality of images produced by each sequence with the available equipment (**Fig. 6**).

DIFFUSION-WEIGHTED IMAGING

The need for diffusion-weighted imaging (DWI) of the bowel is based on the indication for the examination. In those patients undergoing evaluation for suspected bowel malignancy or staging of a known malignancy, DWI should be considered an essential tool for the detection of the primary tumor, solid organ metastases, peritoneal

deposits, and lymph nodes. Quantitative assessment of lesions using the apparent diffusion coefficient value may also be useful for evaluating response to treatment.[45]

DWI for assessment of bowel inflammation, although performed at many institutions, is not universally adopted at this point.[24] There is some evidence suggesting a strong correlation between apparent diffusion coefficient and DWI hyperintensity and the presence of active disease as assessed by disease activity indices.[46–48] These investigations suggest utility for distinguishing active from chronic disease, and DWI may soon become a standard sequence for assessment of inflammatory bowel disease, particularly for those patients who cannot receive intravenous gadolinium contrast.

DWI of the bowel can be performed using either a breath-hold single-shot technique or free

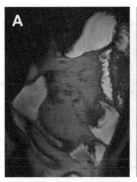
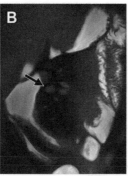
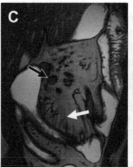
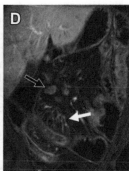

Fig. 6. Coronal SSFSE (*A*), fat-saturated SSFSE (*B*), bSSFP (*C*), and T1-weighted fat-saturated postcontrast (*D*) images demonstrate wall thickening in 2 adjacent loops of ileum in the right lower quadrant of the abdomen. Note the enlarged mesenteric lymph nodes, which are well seen on the fat-saturated SSFSE, bSSFP, and postcontrast images (*black arrows*). The postcontrast and bSSFP (due to chemical shift artifact) images best demonstrate the engorgement of the vasa recta supplying the inflamed segment of bowel (*white arrows*).

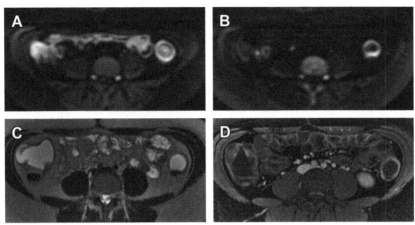

Fig. 7. Axial diffusion-weighted images at b = 500 s/mm² (*A*) and b = 1000 s/mm² (*B*) demonstrate increased signal in the descending colon. Axial SSFSE image demonstrates diffuse thickening of the wall of the descending colon and bright intraluminal contrast throughout the bowel (*C*). The diffusion-weighted image at the higher b value (*B*) demonstrates decreased signal within the fluid-filled loops compared with the lower b value image (*A*). The higher b value results in decreased T2 shine through, which increases the conspicuity of the high signal from impeded diffusion in the wall of the descending colon. (*D*) Axial T1-weighted fat-saturated post contrast image demonstrates enhancement of the wall of the descending colon.

breathing using multiple averages. Free breathing techniques have the advantage of greater SNR and smaller (4–6 mm) section thickness, allowing better correlation with anatomy visible on other sequences.[45] Because the luminal contents can appear bright due to T2 shine-through at lower b values, a b value of at least 800 s/mm² will increase the conspicuity of regions with impeded diffusion (**Fig. 7**).

CINE IMAGING

Cine imaging provides a real-time assessment of bowel peristalsis. Cine imaging can aid in differentiating peristalsing bowel from thickened bowel or stenosis. Cines are usually performed with a coronal bSSFP at a slice thickness of 7 to 10 mm. Images are acquired at 2 images per second for 10 to 20 seconds at each location to cover the entire bowel. Images can be performed during free breathing or during multiple breath-holds. Some investigations suggest that cine imaging may provide increased sensitivity for diseased segments as compared with static imaging alone.[49] In addition, emerging techniques for the quantification of motility suggest that measures of motility may correlate with disease activity.[49,50]

CHEMICAL SHIFT IMAGING

T1-weighted and opposed phase imaging is not commonly used in MR enterography. The utility of this sequence is primarily for the assessment of the solid organs, although it can also aid detection of submucosal fat and mesenteric edema.

Because many patients being assessed for inflammatory bowel disease are relatively young, the likelihood of clinically significant incidental findings for which chemical shift imaging would provide additional information compared with fluid sensitive sequences is thought to be low. Patients that are being imaged for a suspected small bowel tumor, however, may benefit from chemical shift imaging to assess solid organs for primary or metastatic neoplasms.

SUMMARY

MR imaging is increasingly being used for the assessment of the small bowel and colon. Because it does not involve radiation and provides information about both mural disease and extraluminal complications, MR enterography is currently the preferred method for assessing young patients with inflammatory bowel disease. With improving spatial resolution and DWI, MR is also demonstrating utility for screening and assessment of small bowel and colonic neoplasms.

Critical elements for MR imaging of the bowel include sufficient and uniform distension, spasmolysis, and rapid imaging with the appropriate spatial resolution. Each center's protocols for bowel imaging should consider the strengths and weaknesses of the available equipment and the needs of the ordering physicians. With the proper technique, MR of the bowel can provide valuable information about small bowel and colon pathologic abnormality.

REFERENCES

1. Paulsen SR, Huprich JE, Fletcher JG, et al. CT enterography as a diagnostic tool in evaluating small bowel disorders: review of clinical experience with over 700 cases. Radiographics 2006;26(3):641–57 [discussion: 657–62].
2. Duszak R Jr, Kim DH, Pickhardt PJ. Expanding utilization and regional coverage of diagnostic CT colonography: early medicare claims experience. J Am Coll Radiol 2011;8(4):235–41.
3. Panes J, Bouhnik Y, Reinisch W, et al. Imaging techniques for assessment of inflammatory bowel disease: joint ECCO and ESGAR evidence-based consensus guidelines. J Crohns Colitis 2013;7(7): 556–85.
4. Brenner DJ, Hall EJ. Cancer risks from CT scans: now we have data, what next? Radiology 2012; 265(2):330–1.
5. Gupta A, Postgate AJ, Burling D, et al. A prospective study of MR enterography versus capsule endoscopy for the surveillance of adult patients with Peutz-Jeghers syndrome. AJR Am J Roentgenol 2010;195(1):108–16.
6. Patak MA, von Weymarn C, Froehlich JM. Small bowel MR imaging: 1.5T versus 3T. Magn Reson Imaging Clin N Am 2007;15(3):383–93, vii.
7. Adamek HE, Schantzen W, Rinas U, et al. Ultra-high-field magnetic resonance enterography in the diagnosis of ileitis (Neo-)terminalis: a prospective study. J Clin Gastroenterol 2012;46(4):311–6.
8. Shellock FG, Crues JV. MR procedures: biologic effects, safety, and patient care. Radiology 2004; 232(3):635–52.
9. American College of Radiology Committee on Drugs and Contrast Media. ACR manual on contrast media. Version 9. Reston (VA): American College of Radiology; 2013.
10. Svensson MH, Svensson E, Lasson A, et al. Patient acceptance of CT colonography and conventional colonoscopy: prospective comparative study in patients with or suspected of having colorectal disease. Radiology 2002;222(2):337–45.
11. Lauenstein TC, Goehde SC, Debatin JF. Fecal tagging: MR colonography without colonic cleansing. Abdom Imaging 2002;27(4):410–7.
12. Ajaj W, Goyen M. MR imaging of the colon: "technique, indications, results and limitations". Eur J Radiol 2007;61(3):415–23.
13. Achiam MP, Logager V, Chabanova E, et al. Patient acceptance of MR colonography with improved fecal tagging versus conventional colonoscopy. Eur J Radiol 2010;73(1):143–7.
14. Rieber A, Aschoff A, Nussle K, et al. MRI in the diagnosis of small bowel disease: use of positive and negative oral contrast media in combination with enteroclysis. Eur Radiol 2000;10(9):1377–82.
15. Maccioni F, Bruni A, Viscido A, et al. MR imaging in patients with Crohn disease: value of T2- versus T1-weighted gadolinium-enhanced MR sequences with use of an oral superparamagnetic contrast agent. Radiology 2006;238(2):517–30.
16. Laghi A, Paolantonio P, Iafrate F, et al. Oral contrast agents for magnetic resonance imaging of the bowel. Top Magn Reson Imaging 2002; 13(6):389–96.
17. Young BM, Fletcher JG, Booya F, et al. Head-to-head comparison of oral contrast agents for cross-sectional enterography: small bowel distention, timing, and side effects. J Comput Assist Tomogr 2008;32(1):32–8.
18. Lauenstein TC, Schneemann H, Vogt FM, et al. Optimization of oral contrast agents for MR imaging of the small bowel. Radiology 2003;228(1): 279–83.
19. Kuehle CA, Ajaj W, Ladd SC, et al. Hydro-MRI of the small bowel: effect of contrast volume, timing of contrast administration, and data acquisition on bowel distention. AJR Am J Roentgenol 2006; 187(4):W375–85.
20. Siddiki H, Fidler J. MR imaging of the small bowel in Crohn's disease. Eur J Radiol 2009; 69(3):409–17.
21. Darge K, Anupindi SA, Jaramillo D. MR imaging of the abdomen and pelvis in infants, children, and adolescents. Radiology 2011;261(1):12–29.
22. Absah I, Bruining DH, Matsumoto JM, et al. MR enterography in pediatric inflammatory bowel disease: retrospective assessment of patient tolerance, image quality, and initial performance estimates. AJR Am J Roentgenol 2012;199(3): W367–75.
23. Masselli G, Gualdi G. MR imaging of the small bowel. Radiology 2012;264(2):333–48.
24. Ziech ML, Bossuyt PM, Laghi A, et al. Grading luminal Crohn's disease: which MRI features are considered as important? Eur J Radiol 2012; 81(4):e467–72.
25. Thornton E, Morrin MM, Yee J. Current status of MR colonography. Radiographics 2010;30(1): 201–18.
26. Graser A. Magnetic resonance colonography. Radiol Clin North Am 2013;51(1):113–20.
27. Lauenstein TC, Ajaj W, Kuehle CA, et al. Magnetic resonance colonography: comparison of contrast-enhanced three-dimensional vibe with two-dimensional FISP sequences: preliminary experience. Invest Radiol 2005;40(2):89–96.
28. Zijta FM, Nederveen AJ, Jensch S, et al. Feasibility of using automated insufflated carbon dioxide (CO2) for luminal distension in 3.0T MR colonography. Eur J Radiol 2012;81(6):1128–33.
29. Ajaj W, Lauenstein TC, Pelster G, et al. MR colonography: how does air compare to water for

colonic distention? J Magn Reson Imaging 2004; 19(2):216–21.

30. Rodriguez Gomez S, Pages Llinas M, Castells Garangou A, et al. Dark-lumen MR colonography with fecal tagging: a comparison of water enema and air methods of colonic distension for detecting colonic neoplasms. Eur Radiol 2008;18(7): 1396–405.

31. Bakir B, Acunas B, Bugra D, et al. MR colonography after oral administration of polyethylene glycol-electrolyte solution. Radiology 2009; 251(3):901–9.

32. Cronin CG, Lohan DG, Mhuircheartaigh JN, et al. MRI small-bowel follow-through: prone versus supine patient positioning for best small-bowel distention and lesion detection. AJR Am J Roentgenol 2008;191(2):502–6.

33. Grand DJ, Beland M, Harris A. Magnetic resonance enterography. Radiol Clin North Am 2013; 51(1):99–112.

34. Froehlich JM, Daenzer M, von Weymarn C, et al. Aperistaltic effect of hyoscine N-butylbromide versus glucagon on the small bowel assessed by magnetic resonance imaging. Eur Radiol 2009; 19(6):1387–93.

35. Gutzeit A, Binkert CA, Koh DM, et al. Evaluation of the anti-peristaltic effect of glucagon and hyoscine on the small bowel: comparison of intravenous and intramuscular drug administration. Eur Radiol 2012;22(6):1186–94.

36. Lauenstein TC, Ajaj W, Narin B, et al. MR imaging of apparent small-bowel perfusion for diagnosing mesenteric ischemia: feasibility study. Radiology 2005;234(2):569–75.

37. Schindera ST, Nelson RC, DeLong DM, et al. Multidetector row CT of the small bowel: peak enhancement temporal window–initial experience. Radiology 2007;243(2):438–44.

38. Knuesel PR, Kubik RA, Crook DW, et al. Assessment of dynamic contrast enhancement of the small bowel in active Crohn's disease using 3D MR enterography. Eur J Radiol 2010; 73(3):607–13.

39. Pauls S, Gabelmann A, Schmidt SA, et al. Evaluating bowel wall vascularity in Crohn's disease: a comparison of dynamic MRI and wideband harmonic imaging contrast-enhanced low MI ultrasound. Eur Radiol 2006;16(11):2410–7.

40. Vandenbroucke F, Mortele KJ, Tatli S, et al. Noninvasive multidetector computed tomography enterography in patients with small-bowel Crohn's disease: is a 40-second delay better than 70 seconds? Acta Radiol 2007;48(10):1052–60.

41. Rimola J, Ordas I, Rodriguez S, et al. Colonic Crohn's disease: value of magnetic resonance colonography for detection and quantification of disease activity. Abdom Imaging 2010;35(4):422–7.

42. Brauck K, Zenge MO, Vogt FM, et al. Feasibility of whole-body MR with T2- and T1-weighted real-time steady-state free precession sequences during continuous table movement to depict metastases. Radiology 2008;246(3):910–6.

43. Chavhan GB, Babyn PS, Jankharia BG, et al. Steady-state MR imaging sequences: physics, classification, and clinical applications. Radiographics 2008;28(4):1147–60.

44. Rimola J, Ordas I, Rodriguez S, et al. Imaging indexes of activity and severity for Crohn's disease: current status and future trends. Abdom Imaging 2012;37(6):958–66.

45. Sinha R, Rajiah P, Ramachandran I, et al. Diffusion-weighted MR imaging of the gastrointestinal tract: technique, indications, and imaging findings. Radiographics 2013;33(3):655–76.

46. Oto A, Kayhan A, Williams JT, et al. Active Crohn's disease in the small bowel: evaluation by diffusion weighted imaging and quantitative dynamic contrast enhanced MR imaging. J Magn Reson Imaging 2011;33(3):615–24.

47. Buisson A, Joubert A, Montoriol PF, et al. Diffusion-weighted magnetic resonance imaging for detecting and assessing ileal inflammation in Crohn's disease. Aliment Pharmacol Ther 2013; 37(5):537–45.

48. Oussalah A, Laurent V, Bruot O, et al. Diffusion-weighted magnetic resonance without bowel preparation for detecting colonic inflammation in inflammatory bowel disease. Gut 2010;59(8):1056–65.

49. Froehlich JM, Waldherr C, Stoupis C, et al. MR motility imaging in Crohn's disease improves lesion detection compared with standard MR imaging. Eur Radiol 2010;20(8):1945–51.

50. Menys A, Atkinson D, Odille F, et al. Quantified terminal ileal motility during MR enterography as a potential biomarker of Crohn's disease activity: a preliminary study. Eur Radiol 2012;22(11):2494–501.

MR Imaging of the Small Bowel in Crohn Disease

Mahmoud M. Al-Hawary, MD[a],*,
Ellen M. Zimmermann, MD[b], Hero K. Hussain, MD[a]

KEYWORDS

- Crohn disease • Magnetic resonance • Enterography • Inflammation • Fibrosis • Stricture

KEY POINTS

- MR enterography has an established role in evaluating patients with Crohn disease providing essential complementary information to clinical assessment, and as an indispensible adjunct to clinical tools such as colonoscopy.
- MR enterography examinations can establish the diagnosis of Crohn disease, evaluate disease activity and complications, and assess treatment response, thus providing support for clinical decision-making.
- Currently, MR imaging findings are highly predictive of tissue inflammation and can be used clinically to guide clinical care. However, imaging so far has a limited role in accurately identifying stricturing disease.
- Potential exists for MR imaging sequences such as diffusion-weighted imaging and magnetization transfer to assess noninvasively both tissue inflammation and fibrosis and become a highly valuable biomarker of disease progression through monitoring the course of the disease and response to treatment.

INTRODUCTION

Over the past decade, radiologic imaging has come to play an important role in the diagnosis and management of Crohn disease (CD), an inflammatory disease of the gastrointestinal tract.[1] This role in the diagnosis and management was brought about by advances in the radiologic imaging technology and better understanding of the disease process, its natural history, and long-term complications. In addition, the emerging emphasis on mucosal healing as an endpoint in clinical trials, and the potential of potent biologic therapies to alter the natural history of CD, have spurred interest in more complete evaluation of the small intestine. In clinical trials and in clinical practice, optical endoscopy techniques (colonoscopy, deep small bowel enteroscopy, and capsule endoscopy) have been the primary tools used for detecting mucosal inflammation. These techniques allow direct visualization of the intestinal mucosa and the acquisition of mucosal biopsies for histologic evaluation. However, routine colonoscopy has limited ability to access diseased small bowel segments (proximal small bowel disease or proximal to a stenosed ileocecal valve). Furthermore, colonoscopy has drawbacks related to procedural invasiveness including relatively poor patient acceptance, patient discomfort, the need for a bowel preparation, and the risk of bowel perforation.[2] Other diagnostic imaging examinations that are available for the evaluation of CD,

[a] Department of Radiology, University of Michigan Hospitals, 1500 East Medical Center Drive, Ann Arbor, MI 48109, USA; [b] Department of Internal Medicine/Gastroenterology, University of Michigan Hospitals, 1500 East Medical Center Drive, Ann Arbor, MI 48109, USA
* Corresponding author. Department of Radiology, University Hospital, University of Michigan, 1500 East Medical Center Drive, Room B1 D502, Ann Arbor, MI 48109.
E-mail address: alhawary@med.umich.edu

Magn Reson Imaging Clin N Am 22 (2014) 13–22
http://dx.doi.org/10.1016/j.mric.2013.09.001
1064-9689/14/$ – see front matter © 2014 Elsevier Inc. All rights reserved.

including ultrasound, fluoroscopy, computed to-mography (CT), magnetic resonance (MR) imaging, and positron emission tomography with CT (PET-CT), have strengths and weaknesses with respect to small intestinal imaging.[3–5] One particular imaging modality, MR imaging examination, has demonstrated a marked increase in utilization with wider acceptance by both gastroenterologists and radiologists. One of the major advantages driving the increased utilization of MR imaging is the lack of ionizing radiation, an important consideration in young CD patients facing a life-long disease that may require relatively frequent or repeated radiographic examinations. Utilization of MR imaging spares patients the risk of cumulative radiation dose from multiple CT scans.[6–8] Another advantage of MR imaging is the potential for tissue characterization compared with the other imaging techniques given the ability of MR imaging to assess different biophysical characteristics of the imaged tissues (eg, T1-weighting, T2-weighting, T2*-weighting) as well as more recently investigated tissue contrast based on diffusion (diffusion-weighted imaging, DWI) and magnetization transfer (MT).[9–12] The MR imaging examination that is optimized for bowel evaluation is named MR enterography (MRE). In this technique, nonabsorbable oral contrast agent is used to improve bowel distension (eg, polyethylene glycol, mannitol, methylcellulose, or VoLumen [Bracco Diagnostics Inc, Princeton, NJ, USA]) and allow better evaluation of the bowel wall and lumen. The MRE examination allows evaluation of most of the gastrointestinal tract in the abdominal and pelvic cavity (including the stomach, duodenum, small and large bowel down to the anal region) in a single examination, in addition to the evaluation of the extra-enteric abdominal organs.

CD CLASSIFICATION

CD is a chronic transmural inflammatory disorder that can affect any part of the gastrointestinal tract, most commonly the ileocecal region. CD and ulcerative colitis are the 2 major diseases under the umbrella term of "inflammatory bowel disease" (IBD). The inflammatory process in CD patients is thought to arise from altered gut mucosal immunity leading to cytokine overproduction and increased bowel wall leukocyte infiltration.[13] Luminal bacteria and the microbiota likely play a major role in the pathogenesis of IBD. Clinically, the disease is classified into 3 categories as determined by the disease manifestations and symptoms, disease localization in the gastrointestinal tract, and the presence of complications such as strictures or penetrating disease (sinus tract, fistula, or abscess). In the

Vienna classification, disease behavior is separated into 3 prognostic relevant entities including nonstricturing and nonpenetrating (B1), stricturing (B2), and penetrating (B3) disease.[14] This classification system was later modified in the Montreal classification by adding perianal penetrating disease, because perianal fistulas and abscesses have a different prognosis and outcome than intra-abdominal penetrating forms of CD.[15] Patients may remain in the same disease category throughout their life or show disease progression usually from inflammatory to stricturing and penetrating disease. Although these classifications systems were designed originally to classify CD patients for clinical studies, the different subtypes of disease manifestation can be also used to determine treatment decisions. Inflammatory phenotype is treated medically most of the times. The stricturing phenotype requires intervention with mechanical treatments, such as balloon dilatation, stricturoplasty, or resection, in many cases. The penetrating phenotype would eventually require surgical treatment in most cases.[16] MRE can offer similar disease phenotype characterization based on characteristic imaging findings and can differentiate penetrating and stricturing disease from nonstricturing/nonpenetrating (or inflammatory) disease. Accurate disease classification and detection of associated complications on radiologic evaluation are important for guiding the therapeutic decision-making process and has been shown to be better than clinical assessment alone.[17,18] Based on radiologic evaluation and the presence of characteristic findings, bowel involvement can be characterized as active inflammatory, fibrostenotic, or fistulizing/perforating disease, which parallels the clinical classification system.[19] Additional suggested radiologic group is the reparative/regenerative subset, which corresponds to lack of significant disease activity with the presence of mucosal atrophy and regenerative polyps.[19–21] A recent study by Schill and colleagues[22] correlated the behavior assessment performed by a radiologist based on MR imaging findings with the surgeons' clinical assessment based on surgical exploration of patients with CD and found a very high interobserver agreement of 0.937 with identical assessment in 97% of all patients. In a recently published meta-analysis, MR had a per-patient sensitivity of up to 93% in diagnosing IBD,[23] as such MRE examinations are increasingly being used by the gastroenterologists and surgeons as a primary or follow-up imaging modality for assessing disease location and behavior, to decide on further therapeutic options, such as bowel resection, endoscopic or pharmaceutical interventions.[24]

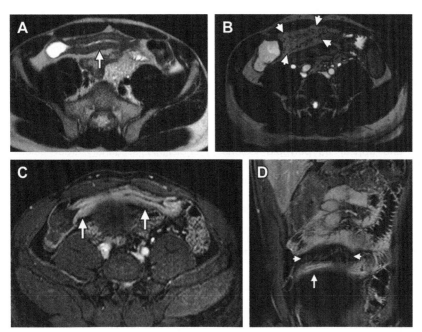

Fig. 1. A 23-year-old male patient with active inflammatory CD. (*A*) Axial T2-weighted single shot fast spin-echo (SSFSE) image demonstrates circumferential bowel wall thickening involving the mid ileum. There is increased signal intensity in the bowel wall indicating bowel wall edema (*arrow*). (*B*) Axial T1/T2-weighted balanced steady-state free-precession (B-SSFP) or balanced turbo field-echo (B-TFE) image demonstrates prominent mesenteric vessels supplying the abnormal bowel segment (*short arrows*). (*C, D*) Axial and coronal T1-weighted contrast-enhanced gradient recalled-echo (GRE) images demonstrate the stratified bowel wall enhancement (*arrows*) with engorged mesenteric vessels (*short arrows*) consistent with active inflammatory disease.

IMAGING FINDINGS

MRE is used to evaluate the entire spectrum of CD manifestations and provide assessment of the disease extent and activity.[25–27] CD evaluation includes both the bowel and the surrounding tissues, as the disease usually starts in the mucosal lining and extends across the bowel wall, potentially involving the peri-enteric structures (mesenteric fat or adjacent organs). Findings related to the bowel seen in active inflammation, includes mucosal ulcerations, a stratified pattern of mural enhancement, and bowel wall thickening (due to edema and infiltration with inflammatory cells) (**Figs. 1** and **2**).[9,19,28] Imaging findings described in fibrostenosing disease include bowel

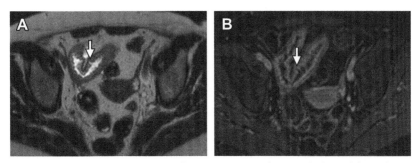

Fig. 2. A 28-year-old female patient with active inflammatory CD and mucosal ulcers. (*A*) Axial T2-weighted SSFSE image demonstrates circumferential bowel wall thickening of the distal ileum with localized areas of deep mucosal ulceration (*arrow*). (*B*) Axial contrast-enhanced T1-weighted GRE image demonstrates stratified bowel wall enhancement and mucosal ulcers (*arrow*) consistent with active inflammatory disease.

wall thickening (due to deposition of collagen), more homogeneous mural enhancement, and luminal narrowing with associated prestenotic bowel dilatation (**Fig. 3**). It is important to note that imaging findings in fibrostenosing disease rely more on lack of findings typically associated with active inflammation rather than direct visualization of fibrotic tissues. Pseudopolyps develop as a consequence of healing, indicate prior severe inflammation, and appear as polypoid lesions seen along the mucosal lining of the bowel. Extension of the inflammation across the serosal lining of the bowel, corresponding to penetrating disease, can lead to formation of a blind ending sinus tract initially, and if there is communication with another structure, a fistula tract develops (eg, enteroenteric, enterocolic, enterocutaneous, enterovesicular) (**Fig. 4**). Penetrating disease can also lead to the formation of adjacent abscess cavity (interloop or perianal) depending on the location of the diseased bowel segment (**Fig. 5**). Additional findings that can be seen in the tissues surrounding the affected bowel segments include reactive enlargement of the mesenteric or pericolic lymph nodes, increased haziness of the mesenteric or per-colic fat due to infiltration by fluid and edema, and engorgement of the mesenteric vessels supplying the affected segment secondary to hyperemia. Fibrofatty proliferation surrounding the affected bowel segments is not specific to disease activity and is usually seen in longstanding disease. Common extraenteric findings include cholelithiasis, urinary tract calculi, and sacroileitis, which can also be assessed on MRE.[29]

INFLAMMATION VERSUS FIBROSIS

One of the primary purposes of radiologic examination in CD is to differentiate active inflammatory from fibrostenosing disease, because this will impact patient management, especially decisions to intensify or optimize immunosuppressive therapies in cases of inflammation, or to intervene early if stricturing or penetrating complications of CD are present.[30] Although imaging findings have shown a strong correlation with tissue

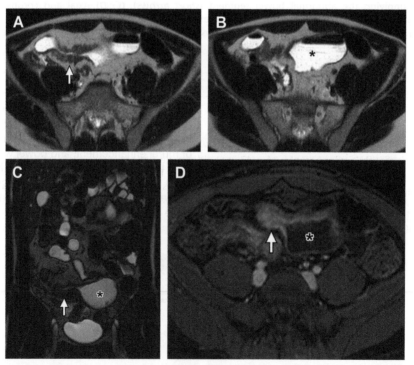

Fig. 3. A 23-year-old male patient with fibrostenosing CD and associated prestenotic bowel dilatation. (*A, B*) Axial T2-weighted SSFSE images demonstrate circumferential bowel wall thickening involving the distal ileum with luminal narrowing (*arrow*) and resultant dilatation of the proximal small bowel (*asterisk*). (*C*) Axial B-TFE image demonstrates a fixed stricture (*arrow*) that persists throughout the study with the prestenotic bowel dilatation (*asterisk*). (*D*) Axial contrast-enhanced T1-weighted GRE image following IV contrast administration demonstrates the homogeneous mural enhancement (*arrow*) with the persistent prestenotic dilatation (*asterisk*) suggesting fibrostenosing disease.

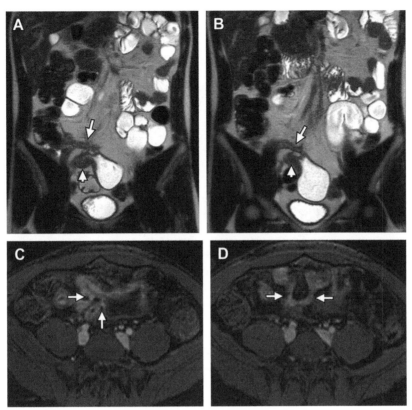

Fig. 4. A 43-year-old male patient with penetrating CD. (A, B) Coronal T2-weighted SSFSE images demonstrate circumferential bowel wall thickening involving the distal ileum with associated luminal narrowing (short arrow) and fistula tracts arising proximal to and at the level of the stricture (arrows). (C, D) Axial contrast-enhanced T1-weighted GRE images demonstrate the enhancing fistula tracts (arrows).

inflammation, the diagnosis of fibrostenosing disease has so far relied more on indirect signs rather than direct tissue characterization. Several studies have shown a strong correlation between disease activity and imaging signs of active inflammation, including stratified mural enhancement of the bowel wall following IV contrast administration, increased T2-weighted signal intensity within the bowel wall indicating edema, haziness of the surrounding mesenteric fat, and engorgement of the peri-enteric vessels.[2,7,31,32] These findings are usually associated with active inflammation in the bowel and are not usually seen in fibrostenosing disease.[33] Rimola and colleagues[2,34] in a prospective study comparing findings on MRE to disease activity on endoscopy showed that the magnitude of quantitative MR changes, such as the presence of bowel wall thickening, bowel wall edema, mural increased signal on T2-weighted imaging, and relative contrast enhancement, closely parallel the severity of bowel lesions detected on endoscopy. They derived a simplified score based on these

MRE findings called the Magnetic Resonance Index of Activity to quantify disease activity in each involved segment. The calculated simplified Magnetic Resonance Index of Activity index was shown to have high (r = 0.81) and significant (P = .001) correlation with the CD endoscopic index of severity in the corresponding segment. In addition, they found mucosal ulcers, enlarged mesenteric lymph nodes, and pseudopolyps to be significantly more prevalent in intestinal segments with more severe endoscopic lesions. More recently, DWI, a widely used biophysical contrast on MR imaging in other organs such as the brain and liver, is being investigated as a noninvasive tool to detect and possibly quantify inflammation within strictures.[11,35] DWI may be used to assess the degree of tissue edema without the need for IV contrast administration and may have a potential role in assessing treatment response or follow-up of patients with known active inflammatory CD (Fig. 6).

In stricturing disease, the longstanding bowel inflammation and tissue remodeling over time

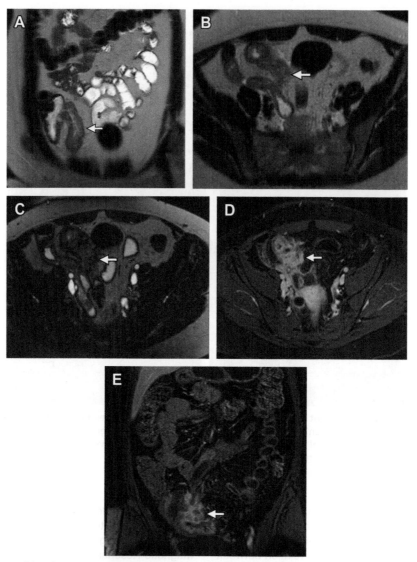

Fig. 5. A 30-year-old male patient with penetrating disease CD and abscess. (*A*) Coronal T2-weighted SSFSE image demonstrates circumferential bowel wall thickening involving the terminal ileum with increased signal intensity in the bowel wall due to edema (*arrow*). (*B, C*) Axial T2-weighted SSFSE and B-TFE images demonstrate stranding of the mesenteric fat proximal to the diseased bowel segment (*arrows*). (*D, E*) Axial and coronal contrast-enhanced T1-weighted GRE images demonstrate multiple enhancing tracts in the same location with a small abscess cavity (*arrows*).

can lead to mural collagen deposition and smooth muscle proliferation resulting in intestinal fibrosis, fixed luminal narrowing, and consequently, in many patients, intestinal obstruction.[36,37] Although endoscopic biopsies, when technically feasible, demonstrate high accuracy for detecting active inflammation, they however only sample the superficial layer of the bowel wall or mucosa and consequently cannot evaluate the deeper bowel wall layers where collagen deposition in stricturing or fibrostenosing disease occurs. In addition, the clinical tools available to assess disease activity, such as optical and capsule endoscopy, serum inflammatory markers such as erythrocyte sedimentation rate and C-reactive protein, endoscopic biopsy grading (CD endoscopic index of severity), and clinical assessment based on the CD activity index, are inaccurate in detecting fibrosis.[38] CD activity index, a commonly used clinical tool to assess disease activity, has been shown to have considerable variation in both the administration and the

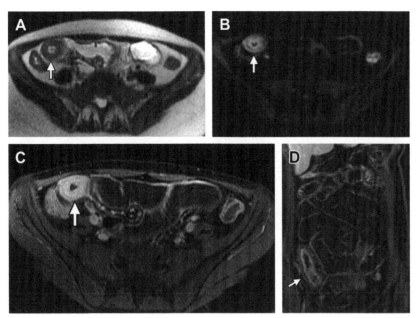

Fig. 6. A 19-year-old female patient with active inflammatory CD. (A) Axial T2-weighted SSFSE image demonstrates circumferential bowel wall thickening in the terminal ileum with increased signal intensity in the bowel wall due to edema (arrow). (B) Axial DWI image (b = 750 s/mm^2) demonstrates increased signal intensity due to impeded diffusion (arrow). (C, D) Axial and coronal contrast-enhanced T1-weighted GRE image demonstrates stratified bowel wall enhancement (arrows) with engorged regional mesenteric vessels indicating active inflammatory disease.

implementation of the score among a pool of experienced researchers and cannot be reliably used.[39] Retrospective evaluation of 18F-FDG-PET/CT, MR enteroclysis, and transabdominal ultrasound could not reliably differentiate inflamed from fibrotic strictures.[40] Similarly, Adler and colleagues[33] have shown that the imaging findings on CTE including mesenteric hypervascularity, mucosal hyperenhancement, and mesenteric fat stranding predict tissue inflammation; however, small bowel stricture without CTE findings of inflammation does not predict the presence of tissue fibrosis. Fibrous strictures often display lack of the classic imaging findings seen in active inflammation, such as high T2-weighted signal in the bowel wall, mucosal ulcerations, and the engorgement of the mesenteric vessels and display a more homogeneous pattern of mural enhancement following IV contrast administration.[41,42] Steward and colleagues[43] showed that the presence of bowel wall thickening and mural enhancement (target sign) correlated positively with the histologic inflammation score; however, this target sign was also a common pattern in fibrostenosis and is seen in 75% of such cases. Consequently, currently available imaging tools do not allow characterization of fibrous tissue and cannot be used solely to determine therapy.

More recently, a promising application of MR imaging has shown potential in assessing the collagen contents of the bowel wall based on the use of the inherent tissue biophysical contrast. Adler and colleagues[12] have investigated the role of MT in detecting intestinal fibrosis in an animal model and found that MT is a promising tool in the identification and quantification of intestinal fibrosis in a rat model of CD. The same group also showed a potential for utilization of MT to assess treatment response and prevention of fibrosis using the same technique.[44] MT imaging was also recently shown to be feasible in humans with sufficient image quality and may help with the identification of fibrotic scarring in patients with CD.[45] Not infrequently, patients with longstanding CD may have coexistent fibrous deposition in the bowel wall in addition to active inflammation corresponding to fibrostenosing disease with superimposed active inflammation, or the mixed type of disease (Fig. 7).[41] Perhaps the best way to describe imaging findings is to report the presence of stenosis with radiographic signs of inflammation versus stenosis without radiographic signs of inflammation. Current MR imaging sequences are highly sensitive to inflammation; however, accurate assessment of tissue fibrosis remains a future aim of this technology.

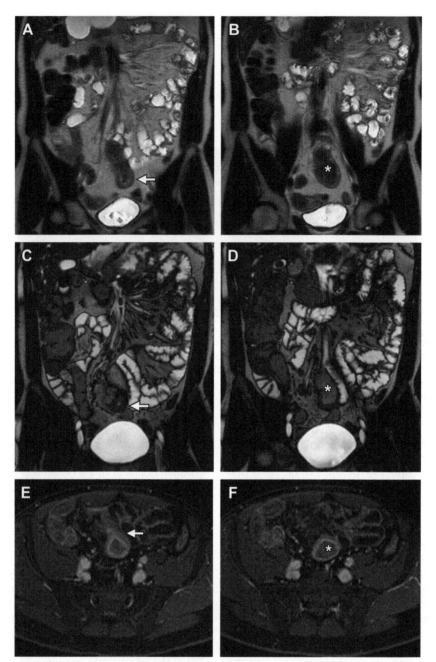

Fig. 7. A 26-year-old male patient with mixed fibrostenosing and active inflammatory CD. (A, B) Coronal T2-weighted SSFSE and (C, D) coronal B-TFE images demonstrate circumferential bowel wall thickening in the ileum, mild increased signal intensity in the bowel wall due to bowel edema (arrow), and proximal bowel dilatation (asterisk). (E, F) axial contrast-enhanced T1-weighted GRE images demonstrate mild stratified mural enhancement with no surrounding fat stranding or prominent regional mesenteric vessels and proximal bowel dilatation (asterisk) suggesting a mixed type disease (arrow).

SUMMARY

MRE has an established role in evaluating patients with CD providing essential complementary information to clinical assessment, and as an indispensible adjunct to clinical tools such as colonoscopy.

MRE examinations can establish the diagnosis of CD, evaluate disease activity and complications, and assess treatment response, thus providing support for clinical decision-making. Currently, MR imaging findings are highly predictive of tissue inflammation and can be used clinically to guide clinical care. However, imaging so far has a limited role in accurately identifying stricturing disease. Potential exists for MR imaging sequences such as DWI and MT to assess both tissue inflammation and fibrosis noninvasively and become a highly valuable biomarker of disease progression through monitoring the course of the disease and response to treatment.

REFERENCES

1. Masselli G, Gualdi G. MR imaging of the small bowel. Radiology 2012;264(2):333–48.
2. Rimola J, Rodriguez S, Garcia-Bosch O, et al. Magnetic resonance for assessment of disease activity and severity in ileocolonic Crohn's disease. Gut 2009;58(8):1113–20.
3. Parente F, Greco S, Molteni M, et al. Imaging inflammatory bowel disease using bowel ultrasound. Eur J Gastroenterol Hepatol 2005;17(3):283–91.
4. Lee SS, Kim AY, Yang SK, et al. Crohn disease of the small bowel: comparison of CT enterography, MR enterography, and small-bowel follow-through as diagnostic techniques. Radiology 2009;251(3):751–61.
5. Shyn PB. 18F-FDG positron emission tomography: potential utility in the assessment of Crohn's disease. Abdom Imaging 2012;37(3):377–86.
6. Tolan DJ, Greenhalgh R, Zealley IA, et al. MR enterographic manifestations of small bowel Crohn disease. Radiographics 2010;30(2):367–84.
7. Gee MS, Nimkin K, Hsu M, et al. Prospective evaluation of MR enterography as the primary imaging modality for pediatric Crohn disease assessment. AJR Am J Roentgenol 2011;197(1):224–31.
8. Jaffe TA, Gaca AM, Delaney S, et al. Radiation doses from small-bowel follow-through and abdominopelvic MDCT in Crohn's disease. AJR Am J Roentgenol 2007;189(5):1015–22.
9. Siddiki H, Fidler J. MR imaging of the small bowel in Crohn's disease. Eur J Radiol 2009;69(3):409–17.
10. Kiryu S, Dodanuki K, Takao H, et al. Free-breathing diffusion-weighted imaging for the assessment of inflammatory activity in Crohn's disease. J Magn Reson Imaging 2009;29(4):880–6.
11. Oto A, Zhu F, Kulkarni K, et al. Evaluation of diffusion-weighted MR imaging for detection of bowel inflammation in patients with Crohn's disease. Acad Radiol 2009;16(5):597–603.
12. Adler J, Swanson SD, Schmiedlin-Ren P, et al. Magnetization transfer helps detect intestinal fibrosis in an animal model of Crohn disease. Radiology 2011;259(1):127–35.
13. Bosani M, Ardizzone S, Porro GB. Biologic targeting in the treatment of inflammatory bowel diseases. Biologics 2009;3:77–97.
14. Gasche C, Scholmerich J, Brynskov J, et al. A simple classification of Crohn's disease: report of the Working Party for the World Congresses of Gastroenterology, Vienna 1998. Inflamm Bowel Dis 2000;6(1):8–15.
15. Satsangi J, Silverberg MS, Vermeire S, et al. The Montreal classification of inflammatory bowel disease: controversies, consensus, and implications. Gut 2006;55(6):749–53.
16. Iesalnieks I, Kilger A, Glass H, et al. Perforating Crohn's ileitis: delay of surgery is associated with inferior postoperative outcome. Inflamm Bowel Dis 2010;16(12):2125–30.
17. Higgins PD, Caoili E, Zimmermann M, et al. Computed tomographic enterography adds information to clinical management in small bowel Crohn's disease. Inflamm Bowel Dis 2007;13(3):262–8.
18. Bruining DH, Siddiki HA, Fletcher JG, et al. Benefit of computed tomography enterography in Crohn's disease: effects on patient management and physician level of confidence. Inflamm Bowel Dis 2012;18(2):219–25.
19. Maglinte DD, Gourtsoyiannis N, Rex D, et al. Classification of small bowel Crohn's subtypes based on multimodality imaging. Radiol Clin North Am 2003;41(2):285–303.
20. Peyrin-Biroulet L, Ferrante M, Magro F, et al. Results from the 2nd Scientific Workshop of the ECCO. I: impact of mucosal healing on the course of inflammatory bowel disease. J Crohns Colitis 2011;5(5):477–83.
21. Daperno M, Castiglione F, de Ridder L, et al. Results of the 2nd part Scientific Workshop of the ECCO. II: measures and markers of prediction to achieve, detect, and monitor intestinal healing in inflammatory bowel disease. J Crohns Colitis 2011;5(5):484–98.
22. Schill G, Iesalnieks I, Haimerl M, et al. Assessment of disease behavior in patients with Crohn's disease by MR enterography. Inflamm Bowel Dis 2013;19(5):983–90.
23. Horsthuis K, Bipat S, Bennink RJ, et al. Inflammatory bowel disease diagnosed with US, MR, scintigraphy, and CT: meta-analysis of prospective studies. Radiology 2008;247(1):64–79.
24. Friedrich C, Fajfar A, Pawlik M, et al. Magnetic resonance enterography with and without biphasic contrast agent enema compared to conventional ileocolonoscopy in patients with Crohn's disease. Inflamm Bowel Dis 2012;18(10):1842–8.
25. Sinha R, Verma R, Verma S, et al. MR enterography of Crohn disease: part 2, imaging and pathologic findings. AJR Am J Roentgenol 2011;197(1):80–5.
26. Sinha R, Verma R, Verma S, et al. MR enterography of Crohn disease: part 1, rationale, technique, and pitfalls. AJR Am J Roentgenol 2011;197(1):76–9.

27. Grand DJ, Beland M, Harris A. Magnetic resonance enterography. Radiol Clin North Am 2013; 51(1):99–112.

28. Costa-Silva L, Brandao AC. MR enterography for the assessment of small bowel diseases. Magn Reson Imaging Clin N Am 2013;21(2):365–83.

29. Smith EA, Dillman JR, Adler J, et al. MR enterography of extraluminal manifestations of inflammatory bowel disease in children and adolescents: moving beyond the bowel wall. AJR Am J Roentgenol 2012; 198(1):W38–45.

30. Hafeez R, Punwani S, Boulos P, et al. Diagnostic and therapeutic impact of MR enterography in Crohn's disease. Clin Radiol 2011;66(12):1148–58.

31. Ziech ML, Bossuyt PM, Laghi A, et al. Grading luminal Crohn's disease: which MRI features are considered as important? Eur J Radiol 2012;81(4): e467–72.

32. Knuesel PR, Kubik RA, Crook DW, et al. Assessment of dynamic contrast enhancement of the small bowel in active Crohn's disease using 3D MR enterography. Eur J Radiol 2010;73(3):607–13.

33. Adler J, Punglia DR, Dillman JR, et al. Computed tomography enterography findings correlate with tissue inflammation, not fibrosis in resected small bowel Crohn's disease. Inflamm Bowel Dis 2012; 18(5):849–56.

34. Rimola J, Ordas I, Rodriguez S, et al. Magnetic resonance imaging for evaluation of Crohn's disease: validation of parameters of severity and quantitative index of activity. Inflamm Bowel Dis 2011;17(8):1759–68.

35. Oto A, Kayhan A, Williams JT, et al. Active Crohn's disease in the small bowel: evaluation by diffusion weighted imaging and quantitative dynamic contrast enhanced MR imaging. J Magn Reson Imaging 2011;33(3):615–24.

36. Rieder F, Fiocchi C. Intestinal fibrosis in inflammatory bowel disease - Current knowledge and future perspectives. J Crohns Colitis 2008;2(4):279–90.

37. Rieder F, Fiocchi C. Intestinal fibrosis in inflammatory bowel disease: progress in basic and clinical science. Curr Opin Gastroenterol 2008;24(4): 462–8.

38. Quencer KB, Nimkin K, Mino-Kenudson M, et al. Detecting active inflammation and fibrosis in pediatric Crohn's disease: prospective evaluation of MR-E and CT-E. Abdom Imaging 2013;38(4): 705–13.

39. Sands BE, Ooi CJ. A survey of methodological variation in the Crohn's disease activity index. Inflamm Bowel Dis 2005;11(2):133–8.

40. Lenze F, Wessling J, Bremer J, et al. Detection and differentiation of inflammatory versus fibromatous Crohn's disease strictures: prospective comparison of 18F-FDG-PET/CT, MR-enteroclysis, and transabdominal ultrasound versus endoscopic/histologic evaluation. Inflamm Bowel Dis 2012; 18(12):2252–60.

41. Rimola J, Rodriguez S, Cabanas ML, et al. MRI of Crohn's disease: from imaging to pathology. Abdom Imaging 2012;37(3):387–96.

42. Oommen J, Oto A. Contrast-enhanced MRI of the small bowel in Crohn's disease. Abdom Imaging 2011;36(2):134–41.

43. Steward MJ, Punwani S, Proctor I, et al. Nonperforating small bowel Crohn's disease assessed by MRI enterography: derivation and histopathological validation of an MR-based activity index. Eur J Radiol 2012;81(9):2080–8.

44. Adler J, Rahal K, Swanson SD, et al. Anti-tumor necrosis factor alpha prevents bowel fibrosis assessed by messenger RNA, histology, and magnetization transfer MRI in rats with Crohn's disease. Inflamm Bowel Dis 2013;19(4):683–90.

45. Pazahr S, Blume I, Frei P, et al. Magnetization transfer for the assessment of bowel fibrosis in patients with Crohn's disease: initial experience. MAGMA 2013;26(3):291–301.

MR Colonography in Inflammatory Bowel Disease

Jordi Rimola, MD, PhD[a],*, Ingrid Ordás, MD[b]

KEYWORDS

- Crohn disease • Magnetic resonance colonography • Colonoscopy • Disease activity
- Inflammatory bowel disease • Ulcerative colitis

KEY POINTS

- MR colonography has a potential role as a complementary or alternative tool to colonoscopy for assessing the extension and severity of activity in inflammatory bowel disease, which is crucial in guiding therapy.
- MR colonography can be performed simultaneously with MR enterography, allowing the activity in both the large and small bowel to be evaluated in a single examination.
- MR colonography has a high accuracy for assessing the activity and severity of Crohn colitis; however, its performance in ulcerative colitis is less clear.
- MR colonography provides accurate information about transmural inflammation and Crohn disease–related complications, such as fistulas or abscesses, which is important for guiding therapy.

INTRODUCTION

In patients with inflammatory bowel disease (IBD), imaging techniques are useful to determine the location, extension, activity, and severity of lesions throughout the course of the disease. The information provided through imaging is crucial for establishing the therapeutic strategy for a particular patient and has prognostic implications.[1]

Conventional colonoscopy is currently considered the reference standard for evaluating disease activity and severity in patients with IBD. However, colonoscopy is sometimes incomplete, and the information it provides is limited to the mucosal surface.

The diagnosis of IBD is based on a combination of clinical, laboratory, and histopathologic data. Therefore, an endoscopic evaluation of the colon and terminal ileum, including multiple biopsies, is needed to diagnose Crohn disease (CD) and ulcerative colitis (UC).[1] However, in CD, lesions not only are confined to the inner wall surface but also involve other intestinal layers and the mesentery. Conventional colonoscopy cannot assess this transmural disease. Furthermore, colonoscopy is not always able to examine the entire colon, and other drawbacks include invasiveness, procedure-related discomfort, risk of bowel perforation, and relatively poor patient acceptance, especially the need for intense colonic cleansing. These disadvantages have led to the search for alternative imaging techniques to assess disease extension and severity in CD, including ultrasound, computed tomography (CT), and magnetic resonance (MR) imaging.[2–4] Although ultrasound is widely available, totally noninvasive, and relatively inexpensive, it is limited by its high dependence on the expertise of the examiner and by the anatomic location of lesions. However, CT is operator-independent but exposes patients to ionizing radiation, limiting its usefulness, especially in younger patients, who must

[a] Department of Radiology, Hospital Clínic Barcelona, CIBER-EHD, IDIBAPS, University of Barcelona, Villarroel 170, Barcelona 08036, Spain; [b] Department of Gastroenterology, Hospital Clínic Barcelona, CIBER-EHD, IDIBAPS, University of Barcelona, Villarroel 170, Barcelona 08036, Spain
* Corresponding author.
E-mail address: jrimola@clinic.ub.es

Magn Reson Imaging Clin N Am 22 (2014) 23–33
http://dx.doi.org/10.1016/j.mric.2013.07.011

be reassessed on multiple occasions over the course of the disease.[5,6]

MR colonography is highly accurate for assessing luminal inflammation, and provides useful information on disease activity, location, severity, and complications, particularly for penetrating and stricturing lesions, which are characteristic features of CD.[4] This information is valuable for guiding medical and surgical treatment and maximizing efficacy and patient safety.

MR imaging has excellent tissular resolution, allowing it to identify inflammation. Unlike CT, MR imaging does not use ionizing radiation, and is associated with a lower incidence of intravenous contrast-related adverse events. Many recent studies have confirmed MR imaging's critical role in assessing patients with CD, not only for evaluating disease activity but also for detecting small bowel lesions and disease-related complications. However, the role of MR imaging in assessing colonic involvement in CD has been investigated less extensively. Recent reports suggest that MR colonography can be useful for evaluating a variety of colonic disorders, including inflammatory diseases.[7-10] MR colonography findings in patients with CD correlate well with those seen at colonoscopy and histopathology, especially for severe lesions.[11,12]

COLONIC LUMINAL INFLAMMATION IN PATIENTS WITH CD

MR colonography findings in CD include ulcers, edema, wall thickening, hyperenhancement after intravenous contrast administration, engorgement of mesenteric vessels (comb sign), enlargement of perienteric lymph nodes, and stranding of mesenteric fat. When assessing activity in patients with CD, one must (1) confirm the presence of mural activity, (2) evaluate the severity of the lesions, and (3) rule out disease-related complications. These 3 aspects are crucial for establishing an optimal individualized therapeutic strategy.[1,3]

Information about disease extension and activity has important prognostic implications and is essential for therapeutic recommendations. Confirmation of luminal activity in a patient with symptoms of a disease flare is crucial in the decision-making process. In 2 large clinical trials, 18% of patients with CD and moderate-to-severe symptoms had no evidence of ulceration at ileocolonoscopy.[13,14] However, another study found that 40% of asymptomatic patients undergoing maintenance treatment with thiopurines had persistent inflammatory lesions.[15]

Intestinal inflammatory changes may be found in various stages simultaneously. A focal patchy discontinuous asymmetrical distribution of abnormalities is a characteristic feature of CD.[16] Some findings of active CD are erosions (aphthoid lesions) and small superficial ulcers.[16] These lesions are easily observed on endoscopic examination but often remain undetected on MR colonography because they are flat.[4,11]

MR colonography findings that correlate with active mucosal and mural inflammation include wall thickening, mural hyperenhancement, mural stratification, edema, ulcers, engorged vasa recta (comb sign), lymph node enlargement, and stranding of perienteric fat (Fig. 1).[17,18] However, systematic reviews of the literature and meta-analyses show that the most frequently used criteria are wall thickening and mural hyperenhancement. Multivariate analyses found that these 2 parameters were independent predictors of activity in different studies.[8,9,19] The per-segment sensitivity of MR imaging in the assessment of colonic activity using these criteria was 70% (95% confidence interval [CI], 67%, 73%), whereas the per-segment specificity was 89% (95% CI, 83%, 96%). However, technical aspects may influence the sensitivity of MR colonography for detecting activity. Indirect data show that MR colonography is generally more accurate when the lumen of the colon is distended. Distending the colon improves the specificity of the technique and also allows better identification of superficial abnormalities, such us ulcerations that can be misread when the lumen is inadequately distended.

Increased wall thickness is observed in bowel segments with active CD. Most authors consider that with optimal luminal distension the colonic wall should be less than 3 mm thick, and any portion of the wall exceeding 3 mm is considered abnormal.[3,4] No agreement exists regarding the normal colonic wall thickness without colonic distension. The degree of bowel wall thickening correlates with both endoscopic and pathologic indexes of CD severity,[9,20,21] and wall thickening only occurs in the late fibrotic stages of the disease. In fact, in the early stages, mural thickening can occur from inflammatory cell infiltration of both the mucosa and submucosa layers. Another common finding in this setting is interstitial edema, which may partially explain wall thickening. Increased mural hyperenhancement is one of the most representative signs of active mural inflammation, even in the absence of wall thickening.[8,9,22] Contrast hyperenhancement can be assessed through comparing thickened bowel segments with adjacent normal loops. The hyperenhancement can be transmural, mucosal, or layered. Whether these patterns of enhancement

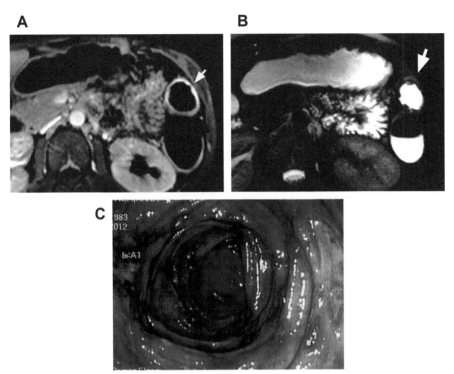

Fig. 1. Luminal colonic CD. (*A*) Fat-saturated T1-weighted image shows wall thickening and mucosal hyperenhancement, which are signs of active inflammation, in the transverse colon. (*B*) Fat-saturated T2-weighted sequence shows edema. Mucosal irregularities corresponding to ulcerations can be detected on both sequences (*arrows*). Conventional colonoscopy also showed severe inflammation (*C*).

have any clinical difference is unclear. Mural hyperenhancement can be explained by the increased number of ectatic capillary vessels in the inflamed bowel wall. Caution is recommended in diagnosing active disease in the setting of suboptimal distension, because the mucosa in these cases may simulate hyperenhancement, leading to erroneous interpretations.[23]

In general, MR colonography studies using negative luminal contrast show a higher accuracy for assessing colonic disease activity.[4] The identification of engorged vasa recta that penetrate the bowel wall perpendicularly, known as the *comb sign*, is an unspecific feature of any inflammatory bowel process, but in the context of CD, it is a marker of colonic segments with active inflammation. This finding is associated with elevated C-reactive protein concentrations.[24,25]

An intrinsic characteristic of CD is that the inflammatory changes may be found in various stages simultaneously, including segments with healing or regenerative changes. Patients with multiple or severe flare-ups may develop postinflammatory pseudopolyps during the regenerative phases in the sites where the inflammation is or was located. These finger-like or polypoid lesions protrude into the colonic lumen. The number of lesions is highly variable, ranging from isolated solitary lesions to multiple lesions with diffuse extension throughout the colon. The adjacent intestinal segments may show signs of inflammation with ulceration or quiescent CD features.[26] Although they have no intrinsic malignant potential, large pseudopolyps can shelter dysplasia or carcinoma,[27] and may be mistaken for neoplastic lesions on both endoscopy and MR colonography.[28,29]

Finally, Oussalah and colleagues[8] evaluated the accuracy of diffusion-weighted imaging (DWI) MR imaging without colonic preparation for assessing colonic inflammation in patients with CD, and found that DWI is nearly as accurate as the MR imaging morphologic findings for detecting activity, but the specificity of the high signal intensity seen in DWI is limited (nearly 60%).

Moderate-to-severe edema can be identified on MR imaging as wall hyperintensity on T2-weighted sequences; however, the absence of this finding cannot rule out active disease. Adding selective saturation of fat signal on T2-weighted sequences increases the sensitivity for identifying edema in the intestinal wall and perienteric fat.

ASSESSMENT OF ACTIVITY AND SEVERITY IN UC

Colonoscopy is the reference standard for evaluating and quantifying disease activity and extent in patients with UC. However, its invasiveness and poor acceptance by patients have prompted, although to a slightly less extent than in CD, the search for alternative or complementary cross-sectional imaging techniques, including MR colonography.

Although MR imaging has proven to be an excellent means of accurately assessing inflammatory changes in colonic CD, its utility in UC has been less extensively evaluated. The first study to indicate the usefulness of MR imaging in assessing UC was published in 1993, wherein wall thickening and hyperintensity of the mucosal and submucosal layers were identified as signs of active disease.[30] Other investigators subsequently confirmed these findings.[30–32]

MR Colonography Features of Activity and Chronicity in UC

UC is a chronic idiopathic inflammatory disease that involves the mucosa of the rectum and colon. Colorectal involvement is one feature that differentiates UC from CD. Characteristically, inflammation spreads proximally from the rectum into the colon to a variable extent in a continuous manner, without skipping areas, and therefore patients progress from proctitis to pancolitis. Rectosigmoid involvement is present in 95% of cases of UC, whereas pancolitis occurs in 35% to 45% of cases. Backwash ileitis is a rare condition (5% of cases) in which the terminal ileum is also involved in the context of pancolitis.[33]

Most MR colonography parameters associated with UC colonic activity were shown to be closely correlated with the severity of endoscopic lesions, and significant differences (P<.001) were found among segments with normal mucosa, mild-to-moderate lesions, and severe disease (except the comb sign, which was similar in mild-to-moderate and severe lesions).[34]

Wall thickening, which is commonly associated with contrast enhancement, is less prominent in UC than in CD, regardless of the degree of severity. Differences in wall thickness between different degrees of severity are usually minimal (range, 1.0–1.2 mm), making simple visual assessment of severity in segments with active UC difficult. However, some patients with severe inflammation may present marked wall thickening.[34–36]

Lastly, the reported rate of ulcers directly identified by MR colonography in UC is much lower (around 35%) than in CD.[34] This difference is probably related to fact that involvement in UC is superficial. The ulcers in UC are usually more subtle than those in CD, and these alterations of the colonic wall are seen as a wavy configuration of the inner wall.[12] In contrast, the outer contour of the wall is usually smoother and more regular in patients with UC than in those with CD, in whom irregular borders are usually seen.

Small amounts of pericolonic free fluid may be seen in cases of severe disease, and this finding indicates focal serosal involvement.[35] Loss of haustra and luminal narrowing are common findings at endoscopy and MR colonography in long-standing inactive disease. Although it is conceivable why the colon wall becomes thickened in a transmural inflammatory disease such as CD, the mechanisms leading to this histologic finding remain unclear in UC, in which inflammation predominantly involves the mucosa. For unknown reasons, in long-standing UC the muscularis mucosa becomes hypertrophied, giving the lumen a typical tubular shape. The submucosa may also have fatty infiltration that contributes to segmental narrowing of some portions of the colon. Fatty proliferation in UC is typically limited to the perirectal space, producing an enlarged presacral space. Less frequently, fatty proliferation can be seen in the sigmoid colon and other colonic segments.[37]

ROLE OF MR COLONOGRAPHY IN DETECTING COLONIC COMPLICATIONS OF IBD

A few studies[18,38,39] examined the usefulness of MR colonography in detecting intra-abdominal colonic fistulas, reporting sensitivities between 71% and 100% and specificities from 92% to 100%. In the only study that reported the results for colonic and small bowel segments separately, the sensitivity, specificity, and overall accuracy of MR colonography were similar for all segments.[38] Fistulas and sinus tracts, hallmarks of CD, are markers of severe disease. Their identification is of paramount importance for several reasons, mainly because the appropriate therapeutic management (medical vs surgical treatment) depends on the adequate characterization of lesions (eg, concomitant abscesses) and because of the prognostic implications for the course of the disease (Figs. 2 and 3).

Tiny fistulas or sinus tracts may be overlooked at colonoscopy because of their size or because the internal orifice is masked by edema.

Abscesses are inflammatory and necrotic collections, usually related to fistula tracts. Abscesses are easily recognized on MR colonography based on their fluid content, with or without gas, circumscribed by a thick enhanced wall. Two studies

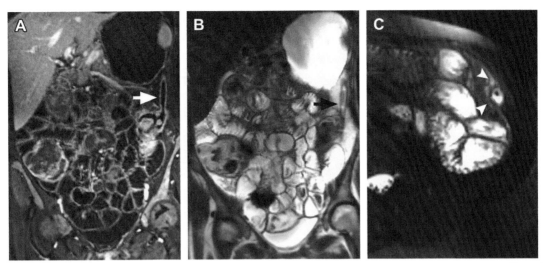

Fig. 2. Penetrating CD in a 35-year-old woman previously diagnosed with CD. Conventional colonoscopy allowed the rectum and sigmoid to be evaluated but could not be completed because of the severity of lesions (not shown). (*A*) Gadolinium-enhanced 3D T1-weighted and (*B*) T2-weighted MR colonographic images show severe inflammatory lesions from the rectum to the transverse colon and a large sinus tract arising from the splenic flexure (*arrows in A and B*). (*C*) Note the inflammatory changes surrounding the sinus tract in the left upper quadrant (*arrowheads*).

evaluated the value of MR imaging in detecting intra-abdominal abscesses in patients with colonic CD, finding sensitivities ranging from 75% to 86% and specificities from 91% to 93%.[18,38]

Colonic distension is crucial for proper identification of colonic stenosis. The impossibility of completing colonoscopic evaluation of the entire colon because of stenosis that precludes the advancement of the endoscope can be overcome with MR colonography, which provides valuable information concerning disease activity and complications in segments proximal to the stenotic lesion. Four studies investigated the accuracy of MR colonography in detecting colonic stenosis in CD, reporting sensitivities ranging from 75% to 100% and specificities from 91% to 100%.[18,20,38,40]

Endoscopic dilation is an effective treatment for stenosis, especially when located in the colon, although improvements in endoscopic techniques are also enabling progressive implementation of this therapeutic option in the small bowel.[41] Because a colonic stricture may impede a complete endoscopic evaluation, MR colonography is extremely useful for characterizing and completing the map of lesions of the unexplored segments; information about the number of strictures and their length and morphology is particularly useful because these characteristics will determine the success of endoscopic dilation. Short strictures may be amenable to endoscopic treatment, whereas longer or curved strictures

cause technical difficulties and may require surgical resection or strictureplasty (**Fig. 4**).[42] When inflammatory and fibrotic components coexist in a single stenotic segment (acute on chronic stenosis), differentiating between them can be challenging because criteria for MR imaging characterization of fibrosis in humans have not been formally defined.

Toxic megacolon is a serious complication of mainly inflammatory or infectious conditions of the colon, commonly associated with UC or colonic CD.[3,33,43] Toxic megacolon is diagnosed through clinical evaluation for systemic toxicity and imaging studies. Colonic dilatation greater than 5.5 cm on plain abdominal radiographs is still the most established radiologic criterion for toxic megacolon. Although the use of MR colonography for providing additional information has not been reported, radiologists should keep this situation and the hallmark features in mind, because some patients may undergo MR colonography as part of the routine assessment of IBD activity and severity (**Fig. 5**).

TOLERABILITY OF MR COLONOGRAPHY IN PATIENTS WITH COLONIC IBD

Bowel cleansing is not strictly mandatory for evaluating inflammatory lesions in the colon, but the absence of residual feces, especially solid feces, improves image quality. However, patients consider bowel purgation the most unpleasant or

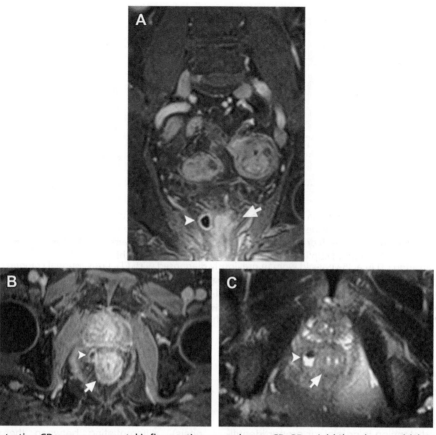

Fig. 3. Penetrating CD on a severe rectal inflammation secondary to CD. 3D axial (*A*) and coronal (*B*) T1-weighted gadolinium-enhanced images show marked mural thickening and mucosal hyperenhancement (*arrows*). A small collection with a rim-enhancing capsule can be identified next to the lower portion of the rectum (*arrowheads*). (*C*) Axial fat-saturated T2-weighted sequence depicts mural edema (*arrow*) and the air-fluid contents of the collection (*arrowhead*).

bothersome part of these procedures.[44–46] Thus, new strategies, such as fecal tagging, have been proposed to obviate bowel cleansing for MR colonography. Fecal tagging is based on altering the signal intensity of stool by adding contrast-modifying substances to regular meals. MR colonography with fecal tagging yielded good results in a study of healthy volunteers,[47] but poor diagnostic accuracy and poor acceptance in a study involving patients.[48] Therefore, fecal tagging must be further optimized, and other strategies, such as intensifying the hydration of stool or low-residual diet prior to MR colonography, must be developed.

MR COLONOGRAPHY AND COLORECTAL CANCER COMPLICATING IBD

Patients with IBD undergo periodic screening colonoscopies for early diagnosis of colorectal cancer lesions. The cumulative incidence of

colorectal cancer in CD is similar to that observed in UC: approximately 1.0% at 10 years, 0.4% to 2.0% at 15 years, and 1.1% to 5.3% at 20 years.[49,50] The carcinomas associated with IBD are often infiltrating and have a poor prognosis.[50]

MR colonography is a suitable modality for detecting solitary polyps and colorectal cancer, but cannot differentiate adenomatous polyps from solitary giant polyps or inflammatory polyps. Considering the underlying inflammatory changes in the intestinal wall that lead to permanent abnormalities, such as pseudopolyps, and the fact that a significant portion of dysplastic lesions are flat at endoscopy, it is conceivable that current cross-sectional imaging techniques would have high rates of false-positive and false-negative diagnoses. MR colonography is not routinely used for colorectal cancer screening in patients with IBD for various reasons. One is that dysplastic lesions in IBD are often flat and only detectable through

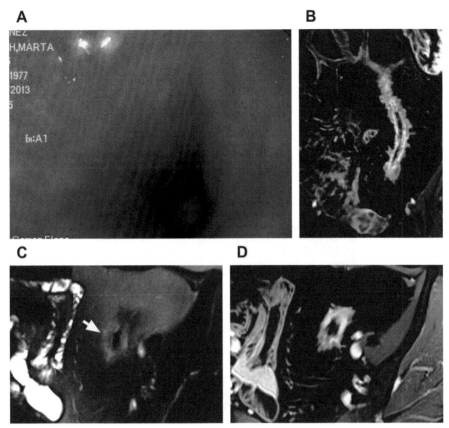

Fig. 4. Stricturing Crohn disease. (*A*) Conventional colonoscopy depicts a normal colonic mucosa with pronounced luminal narrowing at the sigmoid colon. MR colonography confirms the presence of a long luminal stenosis. Both gadolinium-enhanced 3D T1-weighted (*B*) and T2-weighted (*C*) sequences show signs of inflammation: hyperenhancement, wall thickening, and high T2 signal intensity corresponding to edema (*arrow*). Note the fibrofatty proliferation indicating long-standing Crohn disease surrounding the sigmoid (*D*) and the descending colon (*B*). The overall information reported from MR colonography, unavailable from conventional colonoscopy, was key for the proper management of the stenosis.

examining the pit pattern of the mucosa with chromoendoscopy. Another reason is the need for tissue sampling for histologic diagnosis of all suspicious lesions. Therefore, periodic follow-up endoscopy, including chromoendoscopy, is recommended for screening of dysplasia in both CD and UC.[51,52] Nevertheless, MR colonography can be useful in selected cases of incomplete colonoscopy.[3]

PERSPECTIVES OF MR COLONOGRAPHY: CLINICAL PRACTICE AND RESEARCH
MR Colonography in Clinical Practice

Intestinal inflammation in CD can be present in the absence of symptoms and can lead to progressive bowel damage. Impairment of bowel function secondary to CD-related complications may ultimately lead to disability.[53]

Therefore, treatment goals in CD are evolving from mere symptom control toward a more targeted tight control of inflammation. In CD, disease activity can be objectively determined through endoscopic assessment, measurement of biomarkers such as C-reactive protein and calprotectin, and the more recently implemented cross-sectional imaging techniques, especially MR imaging. The information provided by these tools helps clinicians objectively monitor intestinal inflammation, thus increasing the likelihood of achieving treatment goals.[54]

In CD, a careful evaluation of disease characteristics at baseline is crucial to establish the extent, severity, and behavior (inflammatory, stricturing, or penetrating) of the disease. Initial findings provide valuable prognostic information for future follow-up. Therefore, accurate tools should be used for this assessment, not only at diagnosis

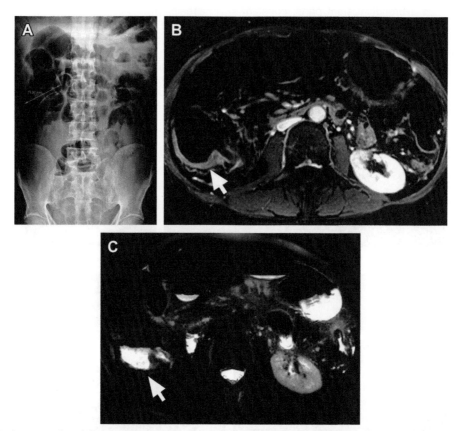

Fig. 5. Toxic megacolon. (*A*) Plain film from a patient with a severe flare of UC shows a marked dilation (>5.5 cm) of the ascending colon, other colonic segments, and the small bowel. (*B, C*) MR imaging without luminal distension acquired the same day also depicts the inflammation over the colon on both gadolinium-enhanced T1-weighted (*B*) and T2-weighted (*C*) sequences (*arrows*).

but also throughout the course of the disease, to optimize and individualize patient management.[55] MR imaging is a valuable tool in this regard, because in addition to accurately corroborating the presence (or absence) of lesions, it also allows complications (stenosis, penetrating lesions) to be ruled out before treatment modification. Endoscopic examination is often incomplete for several reasons. The most frequent are insufficient colonic preparation that precludes a full evaluation of the mucosal surface, and technical difficulties in reaching the cecum and terminal ileum, especially because of impassable stricturing lesions. MR colonography is an accurate method for evaluating colonic CD and can be implemented as an alternative to endoscopy whenever tissue sampling is not required. For all of these reasons, the role of MR imaging in the management of patients with CD will probably continue to expand. The latest consensus guidelines of the European Crohn's and Colitis Organisation (ECCO) and the European Society of Gastrointestinal and Abdominal Radiology

(ESGAR) have incorporated MR imaging as a tool in management algorithms for CD.[3]

MR Colonography in Research: Future Directions

Future roles of MR imaging in the evaluation of patients with CD are expected to include assessment of therapeutic responses, measurement of bowel damage, and assessment of patients in clinical trials.

Along these lines, one MR imaging index of disease activity is an accurate, responsive, and reliable instrument for measuring therapeutic response in CD.[56] Moreover, an ongoing study is aimed at developing a new MR imaging–derived index for measuring structural bowel damage.[53] This instrument will allow the long-term impact of interventional therapeutic strategies on disease outcomes and disease course to be assessed.

Appropriate patient selection for inclusion in trials is of paramount importance for reducing placebo response rates. Centralized review of endoscopic images by expert readers to ensure that patients meet a minimum degree of endoscopic severity has recently been shown to reduce measurement variability and improve statistical efficiency.[57] Centralized MR imaging reading in future clinical trials may help improve patient selection, resulting in more homogeneous populations; more importantly, it may help exclude patients with complications (eg, fistulas and/or abscesses) who would not experience response to therapy or might even experience serious adverse events.

REFERENCES

1. Travis S, Van Assche G, Dignass A, et al. On the second ECCO Consensus on Crohn's disease. J Crohns Colitis 2010;4(1):1–6.
2. Fraquelli M, Colli A, Casazza G, et al. Role of US in detection of Crohn disease: meta-analysis. Radiology 2005;236(1):95–101.
3. Panes J, Bouhnik Y, Reinisch W, et al. Imaging techniques for assessment of inflammatory bowel disease: joint ECCO and ESGAR evidence-based consensus guidelines. J Crohns Colitis 2013;7(7): 556–85.
4. Panes J, Bouzas R, Chaparro M, et al. Systematic review: the use of ultrasonography, computed tomography and magnetic resonance imaging for the diagnosis, assessment of activity and abdominal complications of Crohn's disease. Aliment Pharmacol Ther 2011;34(2):125–45.
5. Chatu S, Subramanian V, Pollok RC. Meta-analysis: diagnostic medical radiation exposure in inflammatory bowel disease. Aliment Pharmacol Ther 2012; 35(5):529–39.
6. Desmond AN, O'Regan K, Curran C, et al. Crohn's disease: factors associated with exposure to high levels of diagnostic radiation. Gut 2008;57(11): 1524–9.
7. Ajaj WM, Lauenstein TC, Pelster G, et al. Magnetic resonance colonography for the detection of inflammatory diseases of the large bowel: quantifying the inflammatory activity. Gut 2005;54(2): 257–63.
8. Oussalah A, Laurent V, Bruot O, et al. Diffusion-weighted magnetic resonance without bowel preparation for detecting colonic inflammation in inflammatory bowel disease. Gut 2010;59(8): 1056–65.
9. Rimola J, Rodriguez S, Garcia-Bosch O, et al. Magnetic resonance for assessment of disease activity and severity in ileocolonic Crohn's disease. Gut 2009;58(8):1113–20.
10. Rodriguez Gomez S, Pages Llinas M, Castells Garangou A, et al. Dark-lumen MR colonography with fecal tagging: a comparison of water enema and air methods of colonic distension for detecting colonic neoplasms. Eur Radiol 2008;18(7): 1396–405.
11. Rimola J, Rodriguez S, Cabanas ML, et al. MRI of Crohn's disease: from imaging to pathology. Abdom Imaging 2012;37(3):387–96.
12. Rimola J, Rodriguez S, Garcia-Bosch O, et al. Role of 3.0-T MR colonography in the evaluation of inflammatory bowel disease. Radiographics 2009; 29(3):701–19.
13. Colombel JF, Sandborn WJ, Reinisch W, et al. Infliximab, azathioprine, or combination therapy for Crohn's disease. N Engl J Med 2010;362(15): 1383–95.
14. Hanauer SB, Feagan BG, Lichtenstein GR, et al. Maintenance infliximab for Crohn's disease: the ACCENT I randomised trial. Lancet 2002; 359(9317):1541–9.
15. Lemann M, Mary JY, Colombel JF, et al. A randomized, double-blind, controlled withdrawal trial in Crohn's disease patients in long-term remission on azathioprine. Gastroenterology 2005; 128(7):1812–8.
16. Kleer CG, Appelman HD. Surgical pathology of Crohn's disease. Surg Clin North Am 2001;81(1): 13–30, vii.
17. Miao YM, Koh DM, Amin Z, et al. Ultrasound and magnetic resonance imaging assessment of active bowel segments in Crohn's disease. Clin Radiol 2002;57(10):913–8.
18. Pilleul F, Godefroy C, Yzebe-Beziat D, et al. Magnetic resonance imaging in Crohn's disease. Gastroenterol Clin Biol 2005;29(8–9):803–8.
19. Rimola J, Ordas I, Rodriguez S, et al. Magnetic resonance imaging for evaluation of Crohn's disease: validation of parameters of severity and quantitative index of activity. Inflamm Bowel Dis 2011;17(8):1759–68.
20. Florie J, Horsthuis K, Hommes DW, et al. Magnetic resonance imaging compared with ileocolonoscopy in evaluating disease severity in Crohn's disease. Clin Gastroenterol Hepatol 2005;3(12): 1221–8.
21. Langhorst J, Kuhle CA, Ajaj W, et al. MR colonography without bowel purgation for the assessment of inflammatory bowel diseases: diagnostic accuracy and patient acceptance. Inflamm Bowel Dis 2007; 13(8):1001–8.
22. Punwani S, Rodriguez-Justo M, Bainbridge A, et al. Mural inflammation in Crohn disease: location-matched histologic validation of MR imaging features. Radiology 2009;252(3):712–20.
23. Lauenstein TC. MR colonography: current status. Eur Radiol 2006;16(7):1519–26.
24. Colombel JF, Solem CA, Sandborn WJ, et al. Quantitative measurement and visual assessment of ileal Crohn's disease activity by computed tomography

enterography: correlation with endoscopic severity and C reactive protein. Gut 2006;55(11):1561–7.

25. Lee SS, Ha HK, Yang SK, et al. CT of prominent pericolic or perienteric vasculature in patients with Crohn's disease: correlation with clinical disease activity and findings on barium studies. AJR Am J Roentgenol 2002;179(4):1029–36.

26. Brozna JP, Fisher RL, Barwick KW. Filiform polyposis: an unusual complication of inflammatory bowel disease. J Clin Gastroenterol 1985;7(5):451–8.

27. Wyse J, Lamoureux E, Gordon PH, et al. Occult dysplasia in a localized giant pseudopolyp in Crohn's colitis: a case report. Can J Gastroenterol 2009;23(7):477–8.

28. von Roon AC, Tekkis PP, Clark SK, et al. The impact of technical factors on outcome of restorative proctocolectomy for familial adenomatous polyposis. Dis Colon Rectum 2007;50(7):952–61.

29. Schottenfeld D, Beebe-Dimmer JL, Vigneau FD. The epidemiology and pathogenesis of neoplasia in the small intestine. Ann Epidemiol 2009;19(1): 58–69.

30. Giovagnoni A, Misericordia M, Terilli F, et al. MR imaging of ulcerative colitis. Abdom Imaging 1993; 18(4):371–5.

31. Madsen SM, Thomsen HS, Munkholm P, et al. Active Crohn's disease and ulcerative colitis evaluated by low-field magnetic resonance imaging. Scand J Gastroenterol 1998;33(11):1193–200.

32. Nozue T, Kobayashi A, Takagi Y, et al. Assessment of disease activity and extent by magnetic resonance imaging in ulcerative colitis. Pediatr Int 2000;42(3):285–8.

33. Stange EF, Travis SP, Vermeire S, et al. European evidence-based Consensus on the diagnosis and management of ulcerative colitis: definitions and diagnosis. J Crohns Colitis 2008;2(1):1–23.

34. Ordas I, Rimola J, Garcia-Bosch O, et al. Diagnostic accuracy of magnetic resonance colonography for the evaluation of disease activity and severity in ulcerative colitis: a prospective study. Gut 2012. [Epub ahead of print].

35. Hafeez R, Punwani S, Pendse D, et al. Derivation of a T2-weighted MRI total colonic inflammation score (TCIS) for assessment of patients with severe acute inflammatory colitis-a preliminary study. Eur Radiol 2011;21(2):366–77.

36. Savoye-Collet C, Roset JB, Koning E, et al. Magnetic resonance colonography in severe attacks of ulcerative colitis. Eur Radiol 2012;22(9): 1963–71.

37. Gore RM. Colonic contour changes in chronic ulcerative colitis: reappraisal of some old concepts. AJR Am J Roentgenol 1992;158(1):59–61.

38. Maccioni F, Bruni A, Viscido A, et al. MR imaging in patients with Crohn disease: value of T2- versus T1-weighted gadolinium-enhanced MR sequences with use of an oral superparamagnetic contrast agent. Radiology 2006;238(2):517–30.

39. Martinez MJ, Ripolles T, Paredes JM, et al. Assessment of the extension and the inflammatory activity in Crohn's disease: comparison of ultrasound and MRI. Abdom Imaging 2009;34(2):141–8.

40. Magnano G, Granata C, Barabino A, et al. Polyethylene glycol and contrast-enhanced MRI of Crohn's disease in children: preliminary experience. Pediatr Radiol 2003;33(6):385–91.

41. Thienpont C, D'Hoore A, Vermeire S, et al. Long-term outcome of endoscopic dilatation in patients with Crohn's disease is not affected by disease activity or medical therapy. Gut 2010;59(3):320–4.

42. Hoffmann JC, Heller F, Faiss S, et al. Through the endoscope balloon dilation of ileocolonic strictures: prognostic factors, complications, and effectiveness. Int J Colorectal Dis 2008;23(7):689–96.

43. Autenrieth DM, Baumgart DC. Toxic megacolon. Inflamm Bowel Dis 2012;18(3):584–91.

44. Thomeer M, Bielen D, Vanbeckevoort D, et al. Patient acceptance for CT colonography: what is the real issue? Eur Radiol 2002;12(6):1410–5.

45. van Gelder RE, Birnie E, Florie J, et al. CT colonography and colonoscopy: assessment of patient preference in a 5-week follow-up study. Radiology 2004;233(2):328–37.

46. Svensson MH, Svensson E, Lasson A, et al. Patient acceptance of CT colonography and conventional colonoscopy: prospective comparative study in patients with or suspected of having colorectal disease. Radiology 2002;222(2):337–45.

47. Lauenstein T, Holtmann G, Schoenfelder D, et al. MR colonography without colonic cleansing: a new strategy to improve patient acceptance. AJR Am J Roentgenol 2001;177(4):823–7.

48. Goehde SC, Descher E, Boekstegers A, et al. Dark lumen MR colonography based on fecal tagging for detection of colorectal masses: accuracy and patient acceptance. Abdom Imaging 2005;30(5): 576–83.

49. Jess T, Rungoe C, Peyrin-Biroulet L. Risk of colorectal cancer in patients with ulcerative colitis: a meta-analysis of population-based cohort studies. Clin Gastroenterol Hepatol 2012;10(6):639–45.

50. Peyrin-Biroulet L, Lepage C, Jooste V, et al. Colorectal cancer in inflammatory bowel diseases: a population-based study (1976-2008). Inflamm Bowel Dis 2012;18(12):2247–51.

51. Farraye FA, Odze RD, Eaden J, et al. AGA medical position statement on the diagnosis and management of colorectal neoplasia in inflammatory bowel disease. Gastroenterology 2010;138(2):738–45.

52. Marion JF, Waye JD, Present DH, et al. Chromoendoscopy-targeted biopsies are superior to standard colonoscopic surveillance for detecting dysplasia in inflammatory bowel disease

patients: a prospective endoscopic trial. Am J Gastroenterol 2008;103(9):2342–9.

53. Pariente B, Cosnes J, Danese S, et al. Development of the Crohn's disease digestive damage score, the Lemann score. Inflamm Bowel Dis 2011;17(6): 1415–22.

54. Peyrin-Biroulet L, Loftus EV Jr, Colombel JF, et al. Early Crohn disease: a proposed definition for use in disease-modification trials. Gut 2010;59(2):141–7.

55. Papay P, Ignjatovic A, Karmiris K, et al. Optimising monitoring in the management of Crohn's disease:

a physician's perspective. J Crohns Colitis 2013; 7(8):653–69.

56. Ordas I, Rimola J, Ripolles T, et al. Accuracy of MRI to assess therapeutic response and mucosal healing in Crohn's disease. Gastroenterology 2011; 140(Suppl 1):140.

57. Feagan BG, Sandborn WJ, D'Haens G, et al. The role of centralized reading of endoscopy in a randomized controlled trial of mesalamine for ulcerative colitis. Gastroenterology 2013;145(1): 149–57.e2.

New Magnetic Resonance Imaging Modalities for Crohn Disease

Joseph H. Yacoub, MD[a], Aytekin Oto, MD[b],*

KEYWORDS

- MR enterography • Crohn disease • DWI • DCE-MR imaging • Small bowel

KEY POINTS

- Three types of sequences constitute a basic magnetic resonance (MR) enterography protocol: single-shot fast spin echo, balanced refocused gradient echo, and fat-suppressed three-dimensional T1 gradient echo.
- High-resolution MR enterography, diffusion-weighted imaging, dynamic contrast-enhanced MR imaging, magnetization transfer, and MR motility imaging are newer techniques that may further enhance the accuracy of MR enterography.
- The goals of imaging in Crohn disease are accurate diagnosis and localization and assessing disease severity, activity, and extent. Assessing disease activity and the presence of penetrating disease have significant implications for the choice of therapy.

INTRODUCTION

Magnetic resonance (MR) enterography is playing an increasing role in the evaluation of the small bowel in patients with Crohn disease (CD). Conventional enteroclysis or small bowel follow-through have been used to evaluate the small bowel; however, with advances in technology, several cross-sectional imaging modalities including computed tomography (CT), MR imaging, positron emission tomography CT, and ultrasound are now available for small bowel imaging. The aim of imaging is to aid in the accurate assessment of the extent, severity, activity, and complications of CD. This role remains the subject of active research with numerous studies and publications in the past decade.[1]

This review article discusses the conventional and emerging MR enterography sequences, and reviews the small bowel imaging findings of CD on MR imaging and the clinical role of MR imaging in the diagnosis of CD and monitoring therapy.

Pathology

CD is an idiopathic, chronic, transmural inflammatory disease that can affect any part of the gastrointestinal tract. It has a tendency toward segmental multifocal distribution. The causes and pathogenesis are not completely understood but are thought to be multifactorial. It is commonly complicated by fistulas, abscesses, bowel obstruction, and neoplasms. CD most commonly affects the small bowel, particularly the terminal ileum. About 70% of patients have small bowel involvement and about 30% have disease limited to the small bowel.[2]

Disclosures: A. Oto, research support from Philips; J.H. Yacoub, none.
a Department of Radiology, Northwestern University, 676 North Saint Clair Street, Suite 800, Chicago, IL 60611, USA; b Department of Radiology, University of Chicago, 5841 South Maryland Avenue, MC 2026, Chicago, IL 60637, USA
* Corresponding author.
E-mail address: aoto@radiology.bsd.uchicago.edu

Clinical Presentation, Evaluation, and Management

The classic presentation of CD is abdominal pain, weight loss, and diarrhea; however, it can have various presentations and tends to have an unpredictable course marked by flares, remissions, and relapses. CD most commonly occurs in early adulthood with a second peak in the elderly. Its diagnosis is based on a combination of clinical findings, endoscopic appearance, biopsy, radiological studies, and/or biochemical markers.[3] Most commonly, ileocolonoscopy and biopsies from the terminal ileum and colon are used to establish the diagnosis. In clinical practice, CD is stratified by disease severity (mild, moderate, or severe), disease location (upper gastrointestinal, ileal, ileocolonic, colonic, or perianal), extent of disease, and disease phenotype (penetrating, stricturing, or inflammatory).[4] Clinical scoring systems have been developed to assess disease severity and activity, the most common of which is the Crohn Disease Activity Index (CDAI), which has been used in many clinical trials; however, it is inconclusive on the severity of the disease.[5,6]

The management of CD is divided into medical therapies and surgical therapies. Therapeutic options are determined by an assessment of the disease location, severity, and extraintestinal complications.[7] Surgery is typically used to treat the penetrating and stricturing complications of CD as well as neoplastic/preneoplastic lesions, suppurative complications, or medically intractable disease.[4,7] Many patients require surgery during the course of the disease; however, surgery is not curative and the disease recurs in most patients within 5 years. Several medical therapies are used in treatment of CD, including corticosteroids, immunomodulators (such as azathioprine, mercaptopurine, and methotrexate), and biologic agents (such as tumor necrosis factor [TNF] alpha inhibitor). The goal of therapy is to induce and maintain symptomatic control, improve quality of life, and minimize short-term and long-term toxicity and complications. A newer goal of therapy is the induction and maintenance of mucosal healing.[7]

MR Enterography Technique

The small bowel is first distended by oral contrast agents. In MR enterography, a large volume of enteric contrast is ingested by the patient over a period of 1 to 2 hours before the onset of the scan. MR enterography is generally preferred to MR enteroclysis because of its comparable performance[8,9] and patient acceptance.[10,11] The most commonly used type of oral contrast agents are biphasic agents that have low T1-weighted signal, which provides good visualization of wall enhancement, and have high T2-weighted signal, which allows assessment of the wall and fold thickness. A spasmolytic agent, such as glucagon, is usually administered before the scan to reduce bowel peristalsis.

Three types of sequences constitute a basic MR enterography protocol: half-Fourier acquisition single-shot turbo spin echo (HASTE), also known as single-shot fast spin echo (SSFSE); balanced refocused gradient echo, also known as balanced steady-state free precession (SSFP), fast imaging using steady-state acquisition (FIESTA), balanced fast field echo (FFE), fast imaging with steady-state precession (true FISP); and postcontrast fat-saturated three-dimensional (3D) T1-weighted ultrafast GRE. In the literature, SSFSE and true FISP sequences are considered complimentary and they are both commonly included in MR enterography protocols. We mostly rely on T2-weighted SSFSE images and, in most cases, have not found true FISP sequences as helpful. In addition to these standard sequences, T2-weighted turbo spin echo (TSE) sequence with fat suppression could be useful to improve the conspicuity of bowel wall edema, but their use is not standard.

Contrast-enhanced images are obtained using T1-weighted ultrafast GRE sequences with fat suppression, which are acquired in 2 or 3 dimensions. The postcontrast images are helpful in evaluating the extent and severity of the disease[12] and are better at visualizing mural stenosis.[13,14] There is no agreement on the optimal scan delay. Inflamed bowel segments enhance early compared with the normal small bowel segments, and enhancement keeps increasing into the delayed phases of 5 to 6 minutes after contrast enhancement. Normal jejunal segments enhance early and more intensely compared with ileal segments. In addition, nondistended small bowel segments may also mimic increased enhancement due to inflammation. One main advantage of MR enterography is that multiple phases of contrasts could be obtained and dynamic contrast enhancement techniques have the potential to provide quantitative parameters to assess wall enhancement and, therefore, disease activity.[15]

ADVANCES IN MR ENTEROGRAPHY TECHNIQUE

High-resolution Images

High-resolution sequences provide the potential for focused evaluation of a small segment of small bowel that is suspected of having disease. In an article by Sinha and colleagues,[16] high-resolution images were obtained of bowel segments that were selected by the radiologist based on suspicion on reviewing the standard sequences. A combination of fat-suppressed true FISP and SSFSE sequences with a small field of view were then obtained. The images were aligned parallel and perpendicular to that bowel segment and were obtained with contiguous thin sections (2–3 mm thick), 160-mm to 250-mm field of view, and a matrix of 128 to 256 by 128 to 256, providing in-plane resolution of 1 to 2 mm. Multiplanar and endoluminal views can then be reconstructed. The investigators reported that this technique increases diagnostic confidence by depicting aphthous ulcers and transmural and mesenteric changes and allows more accurate characterization and classification of CD. In a subsequent study, Sinha and colleagues[17] reported higher accuracy of the high-resolution MR enterography in the diagnosis of bowel ulceration, fistulae, and abscesses using surgical and histologic results as the gold standard. In that study, high-resolution true FISP sequences with smaller fields of view were obtained in each of the 4 abdominal quadrants, adding only 3 minutes to the length of the study. In addition, perpendicular or parallel high-resolution images of involved segments were acquired by the supervising radiologist, if required.

3T Imaging

Imaging with 3-T MR imaging compared with 1.5-T MR imaging increased the signal/noise ratio (SNR) by about 1.7-fold to 1.8-fold,[18,19] which can translate into improving the special resolution or reducing the scan time, both of which would be of particular benefit in the evaluation of the bowel. The T1 shortening effect of gadolinium is more pronounced in 3-T imaging, yielding improved contrast/noise ratio, which translated into increased conspicuity of enhancing structure and lesions, as well as decrease in the amount of gadolinium needed. In addition, fat suppression in 3 T is more pronounced than in 1.5 T because of the wider difference between processional frequencies of fat and water in 3 T.

The advantages of 3-T imaging come at the cost of increasing artifacts and increasing energy deposition.[18–20] Doubling the magnetic field strength quadruples the specific absorption rate (SAR), which becomes a limitation of 3-T imaging, particularly in radiofrequency (RF)-intensive sequences such as SSFSE and true FISP. This effect is particularly relevant in abdominal imaging because the SAR is proportional to the volume being imaged. The increase in SAR can be mitigated by

increasing the recovery time and decreasing the flip angle at the expense of increasing the acquisition time and altering the contrast enhancement. The use of parallel imaging can reduce the number of RF pulses and hence the SAR. In addition, using torso coils instead of body coils can result in a more efficient RF deposition. B1-inhomogeneity artifacts (also referred to as standing wave artifacts or dielectric effects) are local variations in signal intensity across the image that reduce the quality of the image and can obscure certain portions of it by a dark band of low signal. This artifact is more pronounced in 3-T imaging, particularly in wider body habitus, and is even more pronounced in the presence of fluid in the abdomen. This artifact can be reduced by the use of parallel imaging. As an alternative, dielectric pads or RF cushions containing conductive gel could be placed anterior to the abdomen, which was shown to reduce or eliminate the dark B1-inhomogenity artifacts on TSE T2-weighted imaging such as HASTE, but not on true FISP.[21] Chemical shift artifacts of the first type are amplified on 3-T imaging and can be mitigated by increasing the RF at the expense of reducing the SNR. It can also be reduced by applying fat-suppression techniques. Early studies have shown the feasibility of performing high-quality MR enterography on 3 T.[22,23]

Dynamic Contrast-enhanced MR Imaging

Dynamic contrast-enhanced MR (DCE-MR) imaging is being increasingly investigated for quantitative assessment of tissue perfusion. It is most popular in oncologic imaging but increased tissue perfusion is also a hallmark of inflammation. Actively inflamed bowel segments show increased enhancement[12,24–27] with an early hyperenhancement that increases over time until a plateau is reached.[28–31] Bowel that is actively inflamed has also been observed to display a different enhancement pattern and dynamics than inactive disease.[29,32,33] Studies have shown a correlation between dynamic enhancement parameters such as peak uptake and slope of enhancement curve and the clinical activity of the disease[28] as well as inflammatory activity on biopsy.[34,35] Such parameters that describe the enhancement curve (signal vs time) are referred to as semiquantitative analysis. Quantitative DCE-MR imaging analysis has also been applied to MR enterography more recently yielding promising results. In quantitative analysis, pharmacokinetic models are used to convert the signal intensity to the tissue concentration of gadolinium and calculate parameters that reflect the tissue perfusion. The inflamed bowel segments have shown faster values for the transfer constants of the contrast from the intravascular space to the extravascular extracellular space (K^{trans}) and larger volumes of the extravascular extracellular space per unit volume of tissue (V_e).[31]

These semiquantitative and quantitative parameters derived from DCE-MR imaging can be used in distinguishing areas of active inflammation and also have the potential to monitor response following treatment. More efforts to standardize image acquisition and analysis and more studies to confirm the clinical usefulness of these parameters are needed.

Diffusion-weighted Imaging

Diffusion-weighted imaging (DWI) is increasingly becoming a standard part of MR imaging protocols in the abdomen and pelvis. Although most of the literature on DWI has investigated its role in various abdominal malignancies, DWI may likewise have a role as a quantifiable indicator of inflammation. Inflamed bowel segments have shown restricted diffusion compared with normal bowel.[15,36] Oto and colleagues[15] showed that actively inflamed small bowel segments in patients with CD can be differentiated from normal small bowel loops based on DWI and quantitative DCE-MR imaging parameters. The combination of DWI and DCE-MR imaging improved the specificity for detection of active inflammation. Kiryu and colleagues[37] reported a sensitivity, specificity, and accuracy of 86.0%, 81.4%, and 82.4%, respectively, for DWI in the detection of disease-active segments. Restricted diffusion was also shown in inflamed portions of the colon in patients with ulcerative colitis[38–40] and it could be of similar accuracy to contrast-enhanced sequences.[40] In clinical practice, DWI is useful in highlighting bowel segments of active disease and hence it is becoming a standard component of the MR enterography protocol; however, more studies are needed to explore the full potential of this technique and guide its clinical applications. DWI also has the potential to provide quantitative information about the level of inflammation because the apparent diffusion coefficient (ADC) can be calculated from the bowel wall.

MR Motility Imaging Techniques

Real-time images with high temporal resolution (~1–2 seconds) can be acquired by repeatedly acquiring ultrafast true FISP images through a coronal slab of the abdomen to evaluate the small bowel peristalsis. This technique has been referred to as MR motility imaging or cine MR enterography and can be used to identify areas of altered motility, specifically focal areas of paralysis or hypomotility. Froehlich and colleagues[41] detected a larger number of CD-specific findings on cine MR enterography than on static MR enterography alone, and identified significantly more patients with CD than were identified on MR enterography alone. When a change in motility was identified on the cine MR imaging, the corresponding location on the static images was evaluated for CD-specific findings. The CD-specific findings that were analyzed were small bowel wall thickening, stenosis, prestenotic dilatation, layering of the bowel wall (thickened wall combined with alternating hyperintense and hypointense layers within the wall), ulcers, the comb sign, fistulas, and abscess. Kitazume and colleagues[42] described the finding of asymmetric involvement or mesenteric rigidity with antimesenteric flexibility that correlated with longitudinal ulcer in small bowel CD. Software tools for automated evaluation and quantitative analysis of motility on cine MR enterography techniques are only available as research tools and are not yet commercially available.[43,44] Menys and colleagues[44] quantified the motility of the terminal ileum using a new parameter, the motility index (MI), in 28 patients with CD, showing a significant difference in motility between noninflamed and inflamed terminal ileum. The MI was negatively correlated with the acute inflammation score that was assigned to the biopsy, suggesting a role for quantified motility in assessing disease activity.

Magnetization Transfer

One of the most important questions in CD is differentiating between areas of active inflammation that may respond to medical therapy and areas of fibrosis that may require surgical intervention. Most of the current techniques provide, at best, an indirect evaluation of fibrosis, with the recognition that there is significant overlap between fibrosis and inflammation on imaging.[24,45] Magnetization transfer (MT) is a promising MR technique that, in theory, can be used to directly image and quantify fibrosis, differentiating it from edema and inflammation. MT generates contrast that is primarily determined by the fraction of large macromolecules or immobilized phospholipid cell membranes in tissue; stiff body substances such as muscle or fibrotic tissue therefore have a high magnetization transfer effect. In an early study on rats, Adler and colleagues[46] showed that MT ratio correlated with tissue collagen in the bowel but it remained unchanged in control rats that showed inflammation but no fibrosis. Pazahr and colleagues[47] showed that MT imaging of the small bowel wall is feasible in humans if there is sufficient image quality and may help with the identification of fibrotic scarring in patients with CD. The ability to detect fibrosis in small bowel strictures can be useful in choosing between medical therapy in nonfibrotic stenosis and surgical intervention in fibrotic stricture. It can also evaluate response to new therapeutic agents targeted at treating fibrotic strictures.

MR IMAGING FINDINGS OF SMALL BOWEL IN CD

Bowel Wall Findings

Bowel wall thickening (**Fig. 1**) is the most reported imaging finding of CD.[13,48–51] It is best assessed on SSFSE sequence or postcontrast T1-weighted images. The normal bowel wall thickening is 1 to 3 mm, provided the bowel is well distended for evaluation, whereas it typically ranges from 5 to 10 mm in bowel affected by CD.[27] The thickening may decrease in remission, but it is likely to remain thicker than unaffected bowel.[24,27]

Edema in the bowel wall manifesting as increased intramural T2 signal (**Fig. 2**) is one of the most useful finding to indicate active or sever inflammation.[17,24,49,50] Evaluating edema is best done on fat-saturated T2 sequences to differentiate edema from the intramural fat that can be present in chronic CD.

Bowel wall enhancement may be one of the earliest signs of disease activity.[52] It has been repeatedly reported to correlate with bowel inflammation and activity of the disease.[17,27–30,50,51] The pattern of enhancement may be useful in

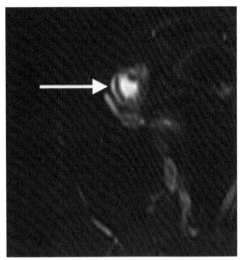

Fig. 2. Small bowel wall edema indicating acute inflammation. A 31-year-old man with CD. Axial T2-weighted fat-suppressed TSE image shows wall thickening with high T2 signal in the wall of the distal ileum (*white arrow*) consistent with wall edema and acute inflammation.

assessing active disease. Homogeneous transmural enhancement (**Fig. 3**) can be seen in active or chronic disease and is therefore nonspecific.[29,50] A layered pattern of enhancement, also known as mural stratification (**Fig. 4**), is more specific for active inflammation.[50,51,53] Bowel wall enhancement has also been observed to decrease in patients transitioning into remission.[27] Restricted diffusion of a bowel segment is another finding suggesting active inflammation in that segment

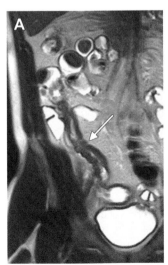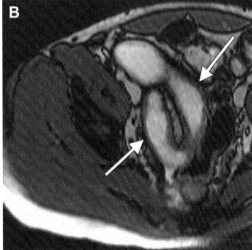

Fig. 1. Small bowel wall thickening. A 35-year-old man with acute-on-chronic CD in the terminal and distal ileum. Coronal HASTE image (*A*) shows wall thickening of the terminal ileum (*white arrow*). Axial true FISP image (*B*) shows wall thickening (*white arrows*) of a bowel segment just proximal to the terminal ileum.

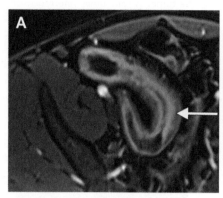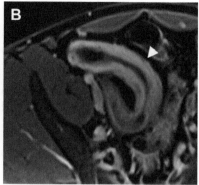

Fig. 3. Increased enhancement of the small bowel wall. A 34-year-old man with CD. Axial fat-suppressed 3D T1 GRE images acquired 50 seconds after intravenous contrast infusion (*A*) and 3 minutes later (*B*) show early mucosal enhancement (*white arrow*) with delayed transmural homogeneous enhancement (*white arrowhead*).

(**Fig. 5**). Hyperintensity on DWI was shown to highly correlate with disease activity evaluated on conventional MR enterography.[54]

Using a high-resolution MR enterography technique, Sinha and colleagues[16] described a new MR imaging finding in CD known as serosal hypervascularity, which is a nestlike lesion of tiny, serpentine enhancing vessels with high signal intensity adjacent to the serosal surface. This finding may predict acute or acute-on-chronic disease.

Mucosal abnormalities, which are hallmarks of CD, are not easily seen on MR enterography. Deep and linear ulcerations may be seen as linear high signal in the thickened bowel wall protruding transversely into the wall (**Fig. 6**) or paralleling the lumen, respectively, provided the small bowel is adequately distended.[13,16] Confluent and intersecting longitudinal and transverse ulcers with residual mucosal islands produce a cobblestone-like appearance. Using high-resolution true FISP sequences, mucosal abnormalities have been depicted with significantly higher accuracy than with standard MR enterography.[13,16,17] In a recent study, the sensitivity and specificity of high-resolution MR enterography for detection of superficial ulcers was 69% and 99%, respectively, and for deep ulcers it was 94% and 99%, respectively.[17] **Fig. 7** shows some of the mural findings of active inflammation in a case of CD involving the colon (see **Fig. 7**).

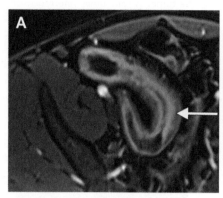

Fig. 4. Layered enhancement of the small bowel wall. A 31-year-old man with CD. Axial, contrast-enhanced, fat-suppressed 3D T1 GRE image reveals a layered enhancement pattern of the wall in the distal ileum with mucosal and serosal hyperenhancement and a region of relative hypoenhancement between the hyperenhancing layers (*white arrows*).

Abnormal Motility

Peristalsis that is abnormally decreased or increased may be an early sign of involvement by active CD that can be identified on MR motility imaging. Froehlich and colleagues[41] classified the abnormal motility based on the pattern of abnormality. If there is no sign of wall movement in the cine sequence it is described as paralysis. A diminished or slow wall movement compared with surrounding bowel sections is described as hypomotility. An increased bowel wall movement compared with surrounding bowel segments is described as hypermotility. In paralysis, the movement of the bowel content would be further evaluated. A to-and-fro movement of the bowel content without any propelling or peristaltic action is described as intraluminal pendular movement. When abnormal motility is identified in any segment, the corresponding location on the static images is scrutinized for additional findings. Using

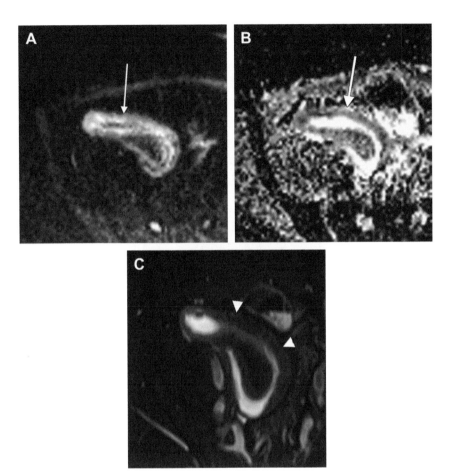

Fig. 5. Restricted diffusion of the small bowel wall. A 34-year-old man with CD. Diffusion-weighted image with b-value of 800 s/mm^2 (*A*) shows high signal in the wall of the distal ileum (*white arrow*) with corresponding dark signal on the ADC map (*B*) consistent with restricted diffusion indicating inflammation (*white arrow*). Axial fat saturated T2-weighted TSE image (*C*) shows the bowel wall thickening corresponding with the diffusion abnormality (*white arrowheads*).

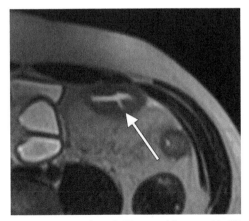

Fig. 6. Transverse ulcer. A 28-year-old man with CD. A linear high T2 signal in the wall of the ileum oriented transverse to the lumen is noted on the axial HASTE image, consistent with a deep transverse ulcer (*white arrow*).

this approach, affected segments were identified that were not detected by static images alone.[41]

Cine MR imaging has also been reported to be useful in detecting abdominal adhesions. Cine views are acquired during Valsalva maneuver and the movement of the bowel loops, or the lack of movement, is observed. The presence of adhesions significantly alters this movement of the bowel loops. Using this technique, good correlations have been reported with surgical assessment in patients without CD.[55,56] The applications of this approach in patients with CD and prior surgeries may be useful in preoperative planning.

Mesenteric Findings

Inflammation of mesentery can point to and confirm disease activity in the adjacent bowel. In addition to stranding of the mesenteric fat, edema,

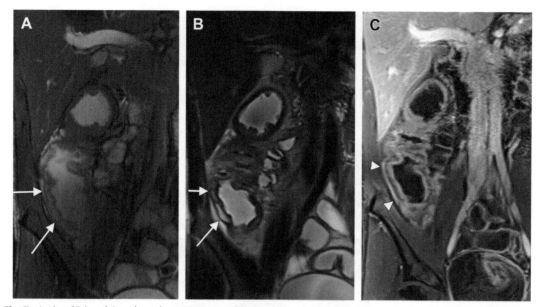

Fig. 7. Active CD involving the colon. A 34-year-old man with a flare of CD and marked active inflammation in the colon. Coronal true FISP (*A*) and coronal HASTE (*B*) images show marked colonic wall thickening with prominent high T2 signal in the wall on the HASTE image consistent with edema (*white arrows*) and active inflammation. Contrast-enhanced coronal fat-suppressed 3D T1 GRE image (*C*) shows layered enhancement pattern of the wall (*white arrowheads*).

and trace free fluid, there are other mesenteric findings that were long recognized in CD and have been shown in MR imaging. The comb sign refers to increased mesenteric blood flow resulting in engorgement of vasculature (**Fig. 8**), which has mostly been reported in active disease.[13,24,52] It is seen on true FISP sequences as low-signal parallel lines, and on contrast-enhanced sequences as parallel lines of enhancement.[13] Mesenteric lymphadenopathy is less specific and can be seen on both active and inactive disease. There is a trend toward higher degree of enhancement of the lymph nodes in active disease,[57] but multiple studies have failed to show a statistical

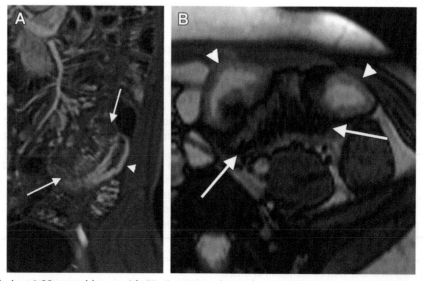

Fig. 8. Comb sign. A 28-year-old man with CD. Contrast-enhanced coronal fat-suppressed 3D T1 GRE (*A*) and axial true FISP (*B*) show engorged vasa recta (*white arrows*), known as comb sign, next to an inflamed enhancing loop of ileum (*white arrowheads*).

difference.[17,24,50] Fibrofatty proliferation around involved bowel loops is a pathognomonic finding in CD that can help to make specific diagnosis in cases with nonspecific bowel inflammation.[58]

Complications

Presence of strictures, fistulas, inflammatory masses, and abscess has major implications on the choice of treatment options and are therefore important to recognize and report. MR enterography has been shown to perform well in depicting mural stenosis, strictures, and obstruction.[13,59] Similar to active inflammation, strictures in CD are also associated with wall thickening (**Fig. 9**). They can cause upstream bowel dilation and obstruction. Fibrotic strictures have low signal on T1 and T2 sequences, and may show low to moderate homogeneous enhancement.

The natural progression of CD disease is from transmural ulceration to extraluminal extension of the inflammation in the surrounding mesentery, which results in sinus tracts or fistulous communications with adjacent bowel loops (**Fig. 10**), organs, or skin. Fistulas appear as linear tracts with high T2 signal with associated enhancement of the tract and surrounding mesentery on the contrast-enhanced sequences.[13,24,60] They can progress into a network of intersecting linear tracts that may tether the adjacent bowel loops. DWI was recently recognized to be particularly useful in detecting fistulas and may be equivalent to post-contrast sequences in the detection of fistulas when combined with a T2 sequence. It can be especially useful in patients with risk factors for contrast agents.[61]

Extension of ulceration into the mesentery may also result in formation of collections of inflammatory tissue (phlegmons) or abscesses. Both are well depicted by MR and appear as heterogeneous lesions with low T1 and intermediate to high T2 signal, with abscesses showing intense peripheral enhancement. DWI can be particularly useful in improving the conspicuity of abscesses.[62]

Patients with CD are at an increased risk for small bowel adenocarcinoma, which may present as a stricture with wall thickening and may be difficult to distinguish form benign strictures. Malignancy is more likely to be associated with focal or segmental mural thickening and mass lesions, whereas benign disease has more generalized and diffuse thickening and an absence of mass.[63]

Perianal Disease

MR imaging is particularly useful in evaluating perianal fistulas and abscesses in CD.[64–67] Fat-suppressed T2-weighted sequences are useful in detecting the fistulas, which appear as bright T2 signal tracts coursing through the para-anal space, ischiorectal fossa, and subcutaneous fat (**Fig. 11**). DWI and contrast-enhanced sequences

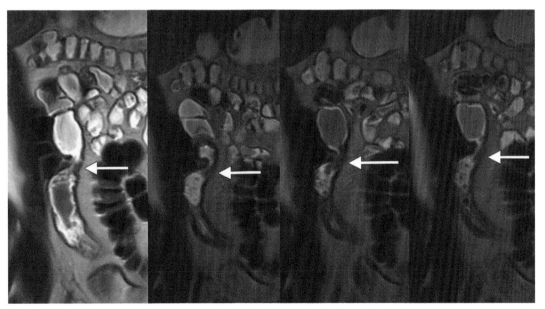

Fig. 9. Focal stricture. A 36-year-old man with CD. Multiple snapshot images at various time points from a true FISP cine sequence (motility sequence) showing a fixed focal narrowing in the ileum (*white arrows*) extending over a length of 2 cm with the lumen measuring 7 mm when maximally open. The bowel loop just proximal to the narrowing is mildly dilated.

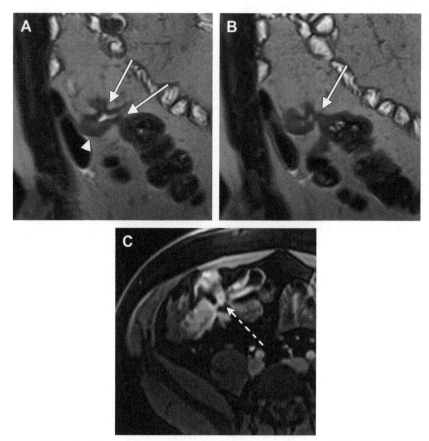

Fig. 10. Enteroenteric fistula. Coronal HASTE images (*A, B*) show complex fistulas involving the terminal ileum, the sigmoid colon, and another loop of ileum with fistulous tract identified from the thickened terminal ileum (*arrowhead*) to each of the 2 other bowel loops (*white arrows*). Contrast-enhanced, axial, fat-suppressed 3D T1 GRE image (*C*) shows a complex fistula causing tethering of the adjacent bowel loops (*dashed white arrow*).

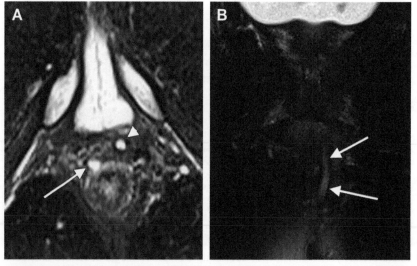

Fig. 11. Perianal fistula. (*A*) Axial fat suppressed T2 TSE image reveals 2 perianal fistulous tracts at the 11 o'clock (*white arrow*) and the 1 o'clock positions (*white arrowhead*). (*B*) Coronal fat suppressed T2 TSE image shows the 1 o'clock tract (*white arrows*) just to the left of midline and anterior to the anal canal (not shown).

are also helpful in detection of fistulas and abscess in the perianal region.[68] The extent of the fistula above the levator ani muscle (ie, into the supralevator space) and the tract course in relation to the internal and external anal sphincters are important factors to report ands have implications for the surgical approach.[66,69] In the surgical classification by Park and colleagues,[70] perianal fistulas are divided into 4 groups based on their relationship to the internal and external anal sphincters in the coronal plane: intersphincteric, transsphincteric, suprasphincteric, and extrasphincteric.[70,71] MR imaging is the best imaging modality to detect and differentiate these different types of perianal fistulas. A study by Horsthuis and colleagues[72] using dynamic MR imaging showed that a faster rate of fistula enhancement correlated with more active disease, suggesting that MR has potential for quantitative assessment of perianal disease activity.

Pearls and Pitfalls

Several pitfalls of MR enterography need to be considered. The normal jejunum enhances more intensely than the ileum; unawareness of this normal enhancement pattern of the jejunum may lead to erroneous overcalling of disease in the normal jejunum. Underdistension of bowel loops can give the false impression of wall thickening and increased enhancement. In contrast, collapsed bowel loops can conceal mucosal findings, such as ulcerations, as well as early strictures. These pitfalls can be avoided be ensuring adequate distention of the bowel. If adequate distention is not achieved, the patient can be given more time to allow the contrast to propagate. As an alternative, additional delayed imaging can be performed. MR motility imaging may also be helpful in avoiding this pitfall, because it allows evaluation of the collapsed segment over time and can therefore help distinguish a fixed narrowing from a lack of distention of a segment.

Wall thickening with homogeneous enhancement can be seen in both active and chronic inflammation. Considering other imaging findings, such as increased intramural T2 signal or layered enhancement, may be more helpful in distinguishing whether active or inactive disease is present. Qualitative and quantitative assessment of DCE-MR imaging may help delineate different patterns of enhancement and has the potential for distinguishing between active and chronic inflammation.

Patients with CD often have a history of prior bowel surgery because of obstructing strictures or severe disease. Postsurgical changes, especially those after a stricturoplasty, may simulate disorders such as strictures or malignancy. Knowledge of prior interventions and review of the concerning segment in multiple planes may be helpful.[73] The use of MR motility imaging may also be useful in detecting postsurgical changes such as adhesion and may improve the delineation between Crohn strictures and postoperative changes.

DIAGNOSTIC PERFORMANCE AND OTHER CLINICAL CONSIDERATIONS

The role of the radiologist starts with providing guidance to the ordering physicians about appropriate studies to order and the imaging techniques available at the institution. Based on a large meta-analysis, the sensitivity and specificity of MR imaging for the detection of CD are 93% and 92.8%, respectively.[1] More recently, Casciani and colleagues[74] reported accuracy, sensitivity, and specificity for the detection of CD of 98.3%, 100%, and 97.6% in a prospective study of 60 pediatric patients. The sensitivity on a per-segment basis may be significantly lower than on a per-patient basis,[75] with reported values varying from 66% to 82% using standard sequences.[17,75] MR enterography is at least of comparable accuracy with conventional enteroclysis[14] and may even detect more abnormalities,[76] particularly in the mesentery,[77,78] although it may be less sensitive for mucosal abnormalities.[77,78] Compared with CT enterography, multiple studies have shown similar sensitivity and specificity.[79–83] The choice between CT and MR enterography at this time is largely affected by the availability of the scanners and the expertise to interpret these examinations.[84]

Some of the accepted indications of MR enterography in CD include (but are not limited to) surveillance of patients with known CD, especially those young in age or who had prior contrast-enhanced CT enterography[85]; evaluation of patients who had incomplete or normal ileocolonoscopy in the setting of clinical suspicion for CD[86]; and as a first-line diagnostic approach in pediatric patients with clinical suspicion for CD.[26,82,87]

One of the main advantages of MR enterography compared with CT or barium studies is the lack of ionizing radiation. This advantage is of particular interest in CD because many patients are young and vulnerable to the effects of radiation.[88] A subset of these patients needs repeated examinations that markedly increase their cumulative radiation dose.[89] In contrast, cost, availability, length of the study, and robustness of the image quality are the disadvantages of MR enterography compared with CT enterography.

The results of MR enterography can have significant impacts on the management of patients with CD. Hafeez and colleagues[90] showed that MR enterography influenced therapeutic strategy in 61% of patients overall and 77% of those with a high underlying clinical suspicion of disease. In another retrospective study of 119 patients at a tertiary referral center for inflammatory bowel disease, MR enterography led to a change in management toward escalation of medical therapy in 55% and surgery in 32.5% of patients.[91] One distinction of major importance to the referring physician is whether there are findings that suggest active inflammation that warrant medical therapy, or whether there is fibrostenotic disease that may require surgical intervention. The presence of stricturing and penetrating disease influences the decision on surgical intervention and its timing. It is therefore important to comment on the presence of penetrating ulcer, sinus tracts, fistulas, inflammatory masses, abscess, and strictures/stenosis while interpreting MR enterography examinations. According to Pozza and colleagues,[92] the presence of an abscess may alter the management to percutaneous drainage, which can facilitate the subsequent surgery or avoid emergency laparotomy. Schill and colleagues[93] showed that MR imaging correlated well with the clinical and surgical evaluation by accurately classifying the disease behavior based on the Montreal classification into 3 categories: nonstricturing and nonpenetrating (B1), stricturing (B2), and penetrating (B3). Ha and colleagues[91] reported that surgical resection specimens corroborated MR enterography findings of disease activity and fibrosis in 92% of cases going to surgery. There is a degree of overlap between active inflammation and fibrosis on imaging that reflects an overlap that is also observed on histopathology.[24,45]

FUTURE CONSIDERATIONS

One of the major interests in MR enterography is its potential role in assessing disease activity. A correlation between MR findings and disease activity has been established.[51,76,94–96] Studies have developed and validated activity scores[94] and quantitative indices based on MR imaging.[49,97] Sempere and colleagues[27] showed that a clinical transition from the active disease phase to remission was associated with a significant decrease in thickness and contrast enhancement of the affected bowel wall on MR imaging. Although the constellation of these studies strongly suggests that MR imaging can assess disease activity, the clinical applications of these findings are not yet completely defined, probably because of the lack of a standardized image acquisition protocol and standardized criteria for assessing disease activity on MR imaging and the lack of a widely accepted algorithm for clinical decision making based on imaging findings.

A potential role for MR enterography in CD is in evaluating response to treatment. In patients with perianal disease, Savoye-Collet and colleagues[98] showed a significant change in MR imaging findings such as hyperintensity on T2-weighted images, and hyperenhancement in patients who responded to the treatment with TNF-alpha inhibitors. In another study by Ng and colleagues,[99] perianal fistulas showed more variable and slower resolution on MR imaging compared with the clinical healing, but, once the healing was seen on MR imaging, the fistula was more likely to remain healed.

Advanced quantitative imaging techniques such as DWI, DCE-MR imaging, quantitative motility, and MT have yet to be applied to clinical practice. In addition to their potential role in assessing disease severity and activity, these parameters may play a key role in monitoring and quantifying the response to treatments, especially disease-modifying therapies such as TNF-alpha inhibitors.

SUMMARY

MR enterography is gaining increased acceptance in the evaluation of CD, but is limited by its availability, cost, and the available expertise. The current technique has already proved to be at least equivalent to other imaging modalities such as CT enterography; however, the addition of functional sequences may provide even more information that could make MR enterography particularly useful in evaluating the activity and severity of the disease and in directing and monitoring therapy.

REFERENCES

1. Horsthuis K, Bipat S, Bennink RJ, et al. Inflammatory bowel disease diagnosed with US, MR, scintigraphy, and CT: meta-analysis of prospective studies. Radiology 2008;247(1):64–79.
2. Martin DR, Lauenstein T, Sitaraman SV. Utility of magnetic resonance imaging in small bowel Crohn's disease. Gastroenterology 2007;133(2):385–90.
3. Van Assche G, Dignass A, Panes J, et al. The second European evidence-based consensus on the diagnosis and management of Crohn's disease: definitions and diagnosis. J Crohns Colitis 2010;4(1):7–27.

4. Cheifetz AS. Management of active Crohn disease. JAMA 2013;309(20):2150–8.

5. Lemann M, Mary JY, Colombel JF, et al. A randomized, double-blind, controlled withdrawal trial in Crohn's disease patients in long-term remission on azathioprine. Gastroenterology 2005; 128(7):1812–8.

6. Colombel JF, Sandborn WJ, Reinisch W, et al. Infliximab, azathioprine, or combination therapy for Crohn's disease. N Engl J Med 2010;362(15): 1383–95.

7. Lichtenstein GR, Hanauer SB, Sandborn WJ. Management of Crohn's disease in adults. Am J Gastroenterol 2009;104(2):465–83 [quiz: 464, 484].

8. Schreyer AG, Geissler A, Albrich H, et al. Abdominal MRI after enteroclysis or with oral contrast in patients with suspected or proven Crohn's disease. Clin Gastroenterol Hepatol 2004;2(6):491–7.

9. Negaard A, Paulsen V, Sandvik L, et al. A prospective randomized comparison between two MRI studies of the small bowel in Crohn's disease, the oral contrast method and MR enteroclysis. Eur Radiol 2007;17(9):2294–301.

10. Negaard A, Sandvik L, Berstad AE, et al. MRI of the small bowel with oral contrast or nasojejunal intubation in Crohn's disease: randomized comparison of patient acceptance. Scand J Gastroenterol 2008;43(1):44–51.

11. Chalian M, Ozturk A, Oliva-Hemker M, et al. MR enterography findings of inflammatory bowel disease in pediatric patients. AJR Am J Roentgenol 2011; 196(6):W810–6.

12. Low RN, Sebrechts CP, Politoske DA, et al. Crohn disease with endoscopic correlation: single-shot fast spin-echo and gadolinium-enhanced fat-suppressed spoiled gradient-echo MR imaging. Radiology 2002;222(3):652–60.

13. Masselli G, Casciani E, Polettini E, et al. Assessment of Crohn's disease in the small bowel: prospective comparison of magnetic resonance enteroclysis with conventional enteroclysis. Eur Radiol 2006;16(12):2817–27.

14. Masselli G, Casciani E, Polettini E, et al. Comparison of MR enteroclysis with MR enterography and conventional enteroclysis in patients with Crohn's disease. Eur Radiol 2008;18(3):438–47.

15. Oto A, Kayhan A, Williams JT, et al. Active Crohn's disease in the small bowel: evaluation by diffusion weighted imaging and quantitative dynamic contrast enhanced MR imaging. J Magn Reson Imaging 2011;33(3):615–24.

16. Sinha R, Rajiah P, Murphy P, et al. Utility of high-resolution MR imaging in demonstrating transmural pathologic changes in Crohn disease. Radiographics 2009;29(6):1847–67.

17. Sinha R, Murphy P, Sanders S, et al. Diagnostic accuracy of high-resolution MR enterography in Crohn's disease: comparison with surgical and pathological specimen. Clin Radiol 2013. http://dx.doi.org/10.1016/j.crad.2013.02.012. [Epub ahead of print].

18. Chang KJ, Kamel IR, Macura KJ, et al. 3.0-T MR imaging of the abdomen: comparison with 1.5 T. Radiographics 2008;28(7):1983–98.

19. Barth MM, Smith MP, Pedrosa I, et al. Body MR imaging at 3.0 T: understanding the opportunities and challenges. Radiographics 2007;27(5):1445–62.

20. Patak MA, von Weymarn C, Froehlich JM. Small bowel MR imaging: 1.5T versus 3T. Magn Reson Imaging Clin N Am 2007;15(3):383–93, vii.

21. Franklin KM, Dale BM, Merkle EM. Improvement in B1-inhomogeneity artifacts in the abdomen at 3T MR imaging using a radiofrequency cushion. J Magn Reson Imaging 2008;27(6):1443–7.

22. van Gemert-Horsthuis K, Florie J, Hommes DW, et al. Feasibility of evaluating Crohn's disease activity at 3.0 Tesla. J Magn Reson Imaging 2006; 24(2):340–8.

23. Dagia C, Ditchfield M, Kean M, et al. Feasibility of 3-T MRI for the evaluation of Crohn disease in children. Pediatr Radiol 2010;40(10):1615–24.

24. Zappa M, Stefanescu C, Cazals-Hatem D, et al. Which magnetic resonance imaging findings accurately evaluate inflammation in small bowel Crohn's disease? A retrospective comparison with surgical pathologic analysis. Inflamm Bowel Dis 2011;17(4): 984–93.

25. Maccioni F, Bruni A, Viscido A, et al. MR imaging in patients with Crohn disease: value of T2- versus T1-weighted gadolinium-enhanced MR sequences with use of an oral superparamagnetic contrast agent. Radiology 2006;238(2):517–30.

26. Laghi A, Borrelli O, Paolantonio P, et al. Contrast enhanced magnetic resonance imaging of the terminal ileum in children with Crohn's disease. Gut 2003;52(3):393–7.

27. Sempere GA, Martinez Sanjuan V, Medina Chulia E, et al. MRI evaluation of inflammatory activity in Crohn's disease. AJR Am J Roentgenol 2005;184(6):1829–35.

28. Pupillo VA, Di Cesare E, Frieri G, et al. Assessment of inflammatory activity in Crohn's disease by means of dynamic contrast-enhanced MRI. La Radiologia Medica 2007;112(6):798–809 [in English, Italian].

29. Del Vescovo R, Sansoni I, Caviglia R, et al. Dynamic contrast enhanced magnetic resonance imaging of the terminal ileum: differentiation of activity of Crohn's disease. Abdom Imaging 2008; 33(4):417–24.

30. Knuesel PR, Kubik RA, Crook DW, et al. Assessment of dynamic contrast enhancement of the small bowel in active Crohn's disease using 3D MR enterography. Eur J Radiol 2010;73(3):607–13.

31. Oto A, Fan X, Mustafi D, et al. Quantitative analysis of dynamic contrast enhanced MRI for assessment of bowel inflammation in Crohn's disease: pilot study. Acad Radiol 2009;16(10):1223–30.

32. Horsthuis K, Bipat S, Stokkers PC, et al. Magnetic resonance imaging for evaluation of disease activity in Crohn's disease: a systematic review. Eur Radiol 2009;19(6):1450–60.

33. Giusti S, Faggioni L, Neri E, et al. Dynamic MRI of the small bowel: usefulness of quantitative contrast-enhancement parameters and time-signal intensity curves for differentiating between active and inactive Crohn's disease. Abdom Imaging 2010;35(6):646–53.

34. Röttgen R, Grandke T, Grieser C, et al. Measurement of MRI enhancement kinetics for evaluation of inflammatory activity in Crohn's disease. Clin Imaging 2010;34(1):29–35.

35. Ziech ML, Lavini C, Caan MW, et al. Dynamic contrast-enhanced MRI in patients with luminal Crohn's disease. Eur J Radiol 2012;81(11):3019–27.

36. Oto A, Zhu F, Kulkarni K, et al. Evaluation of diffusion-weighted MR imaging for detection of bowel inflammation in patients with Crohn's disease. Acad Radiol 2009;16(5):597–603.

37. Kiryu S, Dodanuki K, Takao H, et al. Free-breathing diffusion-weighted imaging for the assessment of inflammatory activity in Crohn's disease. J Magn Reson Imaging 2009;29(4):880–6.

38. Aoyagi T, Shuto K, Okazumi S, et al. Evaluation of ulcerative colitis using diffusion-weighted imaging. Hepatogastroenterology 2010;57(99–100):468–71.

39. Kilickesmez O, Atilla S, Soylu A, et al. Diffusion-weighted imaging of the rectosigmoid colon: preliminary findings. J Comput Assist Tomogr 2009;33(6):863–6.

40. Oussalah A, Laurent V, Bruot O, et al. Diffusion-weighted magnetic resonance without bowel preparation for detecting colonic inflammation in inflammatory bowel disease. Gut 2010;59(8):1056–65.

41. Froehlich JM, Waldherr C, Stoupis C, et al. MR motility imaging in Crohn's disease improves lesion detection compared with standard MR imaging. Eur Radiol 2010;20(8):1945–51.

42. Kitazume Y, Satoh S, Hosoi H, et al. Cine magnetic resonance imaging evaluation of peristalsis of small bowel with longitudinal ulcer in Crohn disease: preliminary results. J Comput Assist Tomogr 2007;31(6):876–83.

43. Odille F, Menys A, Ahmed A, et al. Quantitative assessment of small bowel motility by nonrigid registration of dynamic MR images. Magn Reson Med 2012;68(3):783–93.

44. Menys A, Atkinson D, Odille F, et al. Quantified terminal ileal motility during MR enterography as a potential biomarker of Crohn's disease activity: a preliminary study. Eur Radiol 2012;22(11):2494–501.

45. Al-Hawary M, Zimmermann EM. A new look at Crohn's disease: novel imaging techniques. Curr Opin Gastroenterol 2012;28(4):334–40.

46. Adler J, Swanson SD, Schmiedlin-Ren P, et al. Magnetization transfer helps detect intestinal fibrosis in an animal model of Crohn disease. Radiology 2011;259(1):127–35.

47. Pazahr S, Blume I, Frei P, et al. Magnetization transfer for the assessment of bowel fibrosis in patients with Crohn's disease: initial experience. MAGMA 2013;26(3):291–301.

48. Rimola J, Rodriguez S, García-Bosch O, et al. Magnetic resonance for assessment of disease activity and severity in ileocolonic Crohn's disease. Gut 2009;58(8):1113–20.

49. Rimola J, Ordás I, Rodriguez S, et al. Magnetic resonance imaging for evaluation of Crohn's disease: validation of parameters of severity and quantitative index of activity. Inflamm Bowel Dis 2011;17(8):1759–68.

50. Punwani S, Rodriguez-Justo M, Bainbridge A, et al. Mural inflammation in Crohn disease: location-matched histologic validation of MR imaging features. Radiology 2009;252(3):712–20.

51. Koh DM, Miao Y, Chinn RJ, et al. MR imaging evaluation of the activity of Crohn's Disease. AJR Am J Roentgenol 2001;177(6):1325–32.

52. Fidler JL, Guimaraes L, Einstein DM. MR imaging of the small bowel. Radiographics 2009;29(6):1811–25.

53. Masselli G, Brizi GM, Parrella A, et al. Crohn disease: magnetic resonance enteroclysis. Abdom Imaging 2004;29(3):326–34.

54. Buisson A, Joubert A, Montoriol PF, et al. Diffusion-weighted magnetic resonance imaging for detecting and assessing ileal inflammation in Crohn's disease. Aliment Pharmacol Ther 2013;37(5):537–45.

55. Buhmann-Kirchhoff S, Lang R, Kirchhoff C, et al. Functional cine MR imaging for the detection and mapping of intraabdominal adhesions: method and surgical correlation. Eur Radiol 2008;18(6):1215–23.

56. Lang R, Buhmann S, Hopman A, et al. Cine-MRI detection of intraabdominal adhesions: correlation with intraoperative findings in 89 consecutive cases. Surg Endosc 2008;22(11):2455–61.

57. Gourtsoyianni S, Papanikolaou N, Amanakis E, et al. Crohn's disease lymphadenopathy: MR imaging findings. Eur J Radiol 2009;69(3):425–8.

58. Tolan DJ, Greenhalgh R, Zealley IA, et al. MR enterographic manifestations of small bowel Crohn disease. Radiographics 2010;30(2):367–84.

59. Beall DP, Fortman BJ, Lawler BC, et al. Imaging bowel obstruction: a comparison between fast

magnetic resonance imaging and helical computed tomography. Clin Radiol 2002;57(8):719–24.

60. Rieber A, Aschoff A, Nussle K, et al. MRI in the diagnosis of small bowel disease: use of positive and negative oral contrast media in combination with enteroclysis. Eur Radiol 2000;10(9): 1377–82.

61. Schmid-Tannwald C, Agrawal G, Dahi F, et al. Diffusion-weighted MRI: role in detecting abdominopelvic internal fistulas and sinus tracts. J Magn Reson Imaging 2012;35(1):125–31.

62. Oto A, Schmid-Tannwald C, Agrawal G, et al. Diffusion-weighted MR imaging of abdominopelvic abscesses. Emerg Radiol 2011;18(6):515–24.

63. Fidler J. MR imaging of the small bowel. Radiol Clin N Am 2007;45(2):317–31.

64. Haggett PJ, Moore NR, Shearman JD, et al. Pelvic and perineal complications of Crohn's disease: assessment using magnetic resonance imaging. Gut 1995;36(3):407–10.

65. Laniado M, Makowiec F, Dammann F, et al. Perianal complications of Crohn disease: MR imaging findings. Eur Radiol 1997;7(7):1035–42.

66. O'Donovan AN, Somers S, Farrow R, et al. MR imaging of anorectal Crohn disease: a pictorial essay. Radiographics 1997;17(1):101–7.

67. Schwartz DA, Wiersema MJ, Dudiak KM, et al. A comparison of endoscopic ultrasound, magnetic resonance imaging, and exam under anesthesia for evaluation of Crohn's perianal fistulas. Gastroenterology 2001;121(5):1064–72.

68. Hori M, Oto A, Orrin S, et al. Diffusion-weighted MRI: a new tool for the diagnosis of fistula in ano. J Magn Reson Imaging 2009;30(5):1021–6.

69. Halligan S, Buchanan G. MR imaging of fistula-in-ano. Eur J Radiol 2003;47(2):98–107.

70. Parks AG, Gordon PH, Hardcastle JD. A classification of fistula-in-ano. Br J Surg 1976;63(1):1–12.

71. de Miguel Criado J, del Salto LG, Rivas PF, et al. MR imaging evaluation of perianal fistulas: spectrum of imaging features. Radiographics 2012; 32(1):175–94.

72. Horsthuis K, Lavini C, Bipat S, et al. Perianal Crohn disease: evaluation of dynamic contrast-enhanced MR imaging as an indicator of disease activity. Radiology 2009;251(2):380–7.

73. Sinha R, Verma R, Verma S, et al. MR enterography of Crohn disease: part 1, rationale, technique, and pitfalls. AJR Am J Roentgenol 2011;197(1):76–9.

74. Casciani E, Masselli G, Di Nardo G, et al. MR enterography versus capsule endoscopy in paediatric patients with suspected Crohn's disease. Eur Radiol 2011;21(4):823–31.

75. Dillman JR, Ladino-Torres MF, Adler J, et al. Comparison of MR enterography and histopathology in the evaluation of pediatric Crohn disease. Pediatr Radiol 2011;41(12):1552–8.

76. Frøkjær JB, Larsen E, Steffensen E, et al. Magnetic resonance imaging of the small bowel in Crohn's disease. Scand J Gastroenterol 2005;40(7):832–42.

77. Gourtsoyiannis NC, Grammatikakis J, Papamastorakis G, et al. Imaging of small intestinal Crohn's disease: comparison between MR enteroclysis and conventional enteroclysis. Eur Radiol 2006;16(9):1915–25.

78. Ryan ER, Heaslip IS. Magnetic resonance enteroclysis compared with conventional enteroclysis and computed tomography enteroclysis: a critically appraised topic. Abdom Imaging 2008;33(1):34–7.

79. Jensen MD, Ormstrup T, Vagn-Hansen C, et al. Interobserver and intermodality agreement for detection of small bowel Crohn's disease with MR enterography and CT enterography. Inflamm Bowel Dis 2011;17(5):1081–8.

80. Fiorino G, Bonifacio C, Peyrin-Biroulet L, et al. Prospective comparison of computed tomography enterography and magnetic resonance enterography for assessment of disease activity and complications in ileocolonic Crohn's disease. Inflamm Bowel Dis 2011;17(5):1073–80.

81. Lee SS, Kim AY, Yang SK, et al. Crohn disease of the small bowel: comparison of CT enterography, MR enterography, and small-bowel follow-through as diagnostic techniques. Radiology 2009;251(3): 751–61.

82. Quencer KB, Nimkin K, Mino-Kenudson M, et al. Detecting active inflammation and fibrosis in pediatric Crohn's disease: prospective evaluation of MR-E and CT-E. Abdom Imaging 2013. http://dx.doi.org/10.1007/s00261-013-9981-z. [Epub ahead of print].

83. Grand DJ, Beland MD, Machan JT, et al. Detection of Crohn's disease: comparison of CT and MR enterography without anti-peristaltic agents performed on the same day. Eur J Radiol 2012;81(8): 1735–41.

84. Hafeez R, Greenhalgh R, Rajan J, et al. Use of small bowel imaging for the diagnosis and staging of Crohn's disease—a survey of current UK practice. Br J Radiol 2011;84(1002):508–17.

85. Siddiki H, Fidler J. MR imaging of the small bowel in Crohn's disease. Diagnostic Imaging Inflammatory Bowel Disease 2009;69(3):409–17.

86. Leyendecker JR, Bloomfeld RS, DiSantis DJ, et al. MR enterography in the management of patients with Crohn disease. Radiographics 2009;29(6):1827–46.

87. Gee MS, Nimkin K, Hsu M, et al. Prospective evaluation of MR enterography as the primary imaging modality for pediatric Crohn disease assessment. AJR Am J Roentgenol 2011;197(1):224–31.

88. Palmer L, Herfarth H, Porter CQ, et al. Diagnostic ionizing radiation exposure in a population-based sample of children with inflammatory bowel diseases. Am J Gastroenterol 2009;104(11):2816–23.

89. Jaffe TA, Gaca AM, Delaney S, et al. Radiation doses from small-bowel follow-through and abdominopelvic MDCT in Crohn's Disease. AJR Am J Roentgenol 2007;189(5):1015–22.

90. Hafeez R, Punwani S, Boulos P, et al. Diagnostic and therapeutic impact of MR enterography in Crohn's disease. Clin Radiol 2011;66(12):1148–58.

91. Ha CY, Kumar N, Raptis CA, et al. Magnetic resonance enterography: safe and effective imaging for stricturing Crohn's disease. Dig Dis Sci 2011; 56(10):2906–13.

92. Pozza A, Scarpa M, Lacognata C, et al. Magnetic resonance enterography for Crohn's disease: what the surgeon can take home. J Gastrointest Surg 2011;15(10):1689–98.

93. Schill G, Iesalnieks I, Haimerl M, et al. Assessment of disease behavior in patients with Crohn's disease by MR enterography. Inflamm Bowel Dis 2013;19(5):983–90.

94. Girometti R, Zuiani C, Toso F, et al. MRI scoring system including dynamic motility evaluation in assessing the activity of Crohn's disease of the terminal ileum. Acad Radiol 2008;15(2):153–64.

95. Albert JG, Martiny F, Krummenerl A, et al. Diagnosis of small bowel Crohn's disease: a prospective comparison of capsule endoscopy with magnetic resonance imaging and fluoroscopic enteroclysis. Gut 2005;54(12):1721–7.

96. Maccioni F, Viscido A, Broglia L, et al. Evaluation of Crohn disease activity with magnetic resonance imaging. Abdom Imaging 2000;25(3):219–28.

97. Steward MJ, Punwani S, Proctor I, et al. Non-perforating small bowel Crohn's disease assessed by MRI enterography: derivation and histopathological validation of an MR-based activity index. Eur J Radiol 2012;81(9):2080–8.

98. Savoye-Collet C, Savoye G, Koning E, et al. Fistulizing perianal Crohn's disease: contrast-enhanced magnetic resonance imaging assessment at 1 year on maintenance anti-TNF-alpha therapy. Inflamm Bowel Dis 2011;17(8):1751–8.

99. Ng SC, Plamondon S, Gupta A, et al. Prospective evaluation of anti-tumor necrosis factor therapy guided by magnetic resonance imaging for Crohn's perineal fistulas. Am J Gastroenterol 2009;104(12):2973–86.

Noninflammatory Conditions of the Small Bowel

Gabriele Masselli, MD*, Elisabetta Polettini, MD,
Francesca Laghi, MD, Riccardo Monti, MD,
Gianfranco Gualdi, MD

KEYWORDS

- Magnetic resonance imaging • Small bowel • Neoplasm • Enteroclysis • Enterography
- Obstruction

KEY POINTS

- Magnetic resonance (MR) enteroclysis provides adequate distension of the entire small bowel and can exclude small-bowel disease reliably.
- MR enteroclysis is an effective diagnostic technique in patients suspected of having small-bowel neoplasms.
- MR enteroclysis may also be used to distinguish neoplasms from inflammatory diseases.
- Small polypoid masses that do not cause an obstruction may be difficult to detect using MR enterography.
- Intraintestinal and extraintestinal features detected with MR imaging may be helpful in establishing a diagnosis of celiac disease and in clarifying the causes of nonspecific gastrointestinal symptoms in patients with previously undiagnosed celiac disease.

INTRODUCTION

Tumors of the small bowel are infrequent, accounting for about 3% to 6% of all gastrointestinal (GI) neoplasms. Diagnosis is not easy, owing to the nonspecific symptoms and because the mesenteric small bowel is traditionally the most difficult portion of the GI tract to investigate.

Most tumors are not determined by obstruction, and very often manifest with obscure GI bleeding, anemia, and abdominal pain. In the case of neuroendocrine tumors, the clinical manifestation depends on the hormones produced by the tumors.

Conventional enteroclysis and capsule endoscopy are the procedures most commonly used to visualize mucosal abnormalities, but are limited in the evaluation of mural and extramural extent of small-bowel tumors.[1,2] Therefore, radiologists assume a major role in the detection of small-bowel tumors. However, inadequate radiologic studies may cause incorrect interpretation of radiologic findings, leading to crucial delay in diagnosing primary malignancies of the small intestine.

Magnetic resonance (MR) imaging has a leading role in the diagnosis not only of tumors but also of many diseases of the small intestine. The lack of ionizing radiation, the possibility of combining the morphologic information of cross-sectional imaging with functional information, the excellent soft-tissue contrast, and a relatively safe intravenous contrast agent profile make MR imaging the method of choice for the study of the small intestine. Moreover, the opportunity of studying surrounding structures (eg, for detection of any metastases in the liver) make MR imaging an excellent method not only for diagnosis but also for staging and prognosis. The intraluminal and extraluminal MR findings, combined with contrast enhancement and functional information, help to make an accurate diagnosis and, consequently, characterize small-bowel neoplasms.

Radiology Department, Umberto I hospital, Sapienza University, Via del Policlinico 155, Rome 00161, Italy
* Corresponding author.
E-mail address: g.masselli@policlinicoumberto1.it

Magn Reson Imaging Clin N Am 22 (2014) 51–65
http://dx.doi.org/10.1016/j.mric.2013.07.012

mri.theclinics.com

Celiac disease is characterized by malabsorption of the intestine, which develops as a result of gluten and/or gluten-related protein intake. MR imaging provides morphologic information obtained noninvasively, such as fold pattern abnormalities and bowel dilatation, as well as extraintestinal findings such as mesenteric vascular congestion, lymphadenopathy, hyposplenism, and intussusception.

This article describes MR findings of primary small-bowel neoplasms and celiac disease, and discusses MR findings for the differential diagnosis.

TECHNICAL CONSIDERATIONS
Contrast Agents

A substance to be considered a good enteral agent should guarantee uniform and homogeneous opacification, adequate distension of small-bowel lumen, high contrast between the lumen and the small bowel, low cost, and the absence of serious adverse side effects.

A several number of enteral agents have been proposed for use in MR imaging of the small bowel. All of these substances are classified according to the intensity produced: positive, negative, or biphasic contrast enteral agents.

Positive contrast enteral agents have high signal intensity on T1-weighted images; gadolinium chelates,[3] manganese ions,[4] ferrous ions,[5] and foods such as blueberry juice[6] belong to this group. Using these contrast agents it is possible to show wall thickening on T1-weighted images; their limitation is the detection of more subtle mucosal or wall hyperenhancement after the intravenous injection of gadolinium-based contrast material.

Negative contrast enteral agents have low signal intensity on T2-weighted images. These agents constitute solutions with superparamagnetic iron oxides (SPIOs), including nanoparticles of maghemite in bentonite matrix, and ultrasmall SPIOs (USPIOs).[7] On T2-weighted images, the inflammation in the bowel wall is much more pronounced because negative contrast agents reduce the signal intensity of the bowel lumen.

However, the low signal intensity of intraluminal contrast on T2-weighted images and the associated susceptibility effects may reduce the conspicuity of the normal small-bowel wall and of low–signal-intensity lesions, such as carcinoid tumors, as well as of intraluminal abnormalities.

For suspected small-bowel neoplasms it is recommended to use biphasic agents, such as water, Volumen, sorbitol, and polyethylene glycol (PEG), which produce low signal intensity on T1-weighted images and high signal intensity on T2-weighted images. These agents provide conspicuous distinction between the bowel wall and the lumen, both on T2-weighted images (eg, by enabling the detection of mural ulcers, which could otherwise be missed, being darkened if a negative—hypointense—contrast agent is used) and on T1-weighted postgadolinium images (eg, by increasing the conspicuity of hyperenhancing masses).

On T1-weighted images, the contrast between the bowel lumen and masses after intravenous administration of contrast material is increased. The high contrast between the lumen and the dark bowel wall on T2-weighted images improves the detection of endoluminal abnormalities and more effectively highlights transmural ulcers.[8,9]

The role of gadolinium chelates for the detection of small-bowel tumors has yet to be clearly defined. The accuracy of a nonenhanced MR protocol designed for detection of small-intestinal neoplasms was recently found to be similar to that of a protocol that included contrast enhancement.[2,10]

Gadolinium-enhanced fat-saturated T1-weighted pulse sequences help to characterize small-bowel tumors because of their enhancement pattern, and to stage neoplasms by evaluating the presence of liver and mesenteric metastasis.[9,11,12] Moreover, the use of gadolinium-enhanced T1-weighted sequences allows the characterization of malignant versus benign strictures in small-bowel obstruction.[13]

Contrast-enhanced sequences help to differentiate inflammatory from noninflammatory diseases, thereby increasing diagnostic accuracy. Dynamic contrast-enhanced MR imaging of the small bowel may be useful in evaluating and identifying bowel-wall inflammation in patients with celiac disease.

The use of gadolinium is highly discouraged in pregnant patients and in patients with renal failure, as it increases the risk of developing nephrogenic systemic fibrosis.

MR Techniques: Enterography and Enteroclysis

The first step in the evaluation of the small intestine is to achieve a good distension of the small bowels. This distension is critical because collapsed bowel loops may hide lesions or mimic disease by mistakenly suggesting that the collapsed segments are actually an abnormality-related thickened bowel wall.[14]

At present there are 2 basic methods to obtain distension of the small bowel, namely MR enteroclysis and MR enterography; the first is obtained by infusion of the contrast material through a nasojejunal tube, the second by oral administration of contrast material.[15,16]

The choice between the intubation-infusion method (enteroclysis) and the oral approach (enterography) is controversial and depends on the clinical indications, the patient population, the radiology practice, and the diagnostic algorithms of different centers.[17,18]

Enteroclysis is reported to be the only method that invariably provides adequate distension of the entire small bowel, and can help exclude small-bowel disease reliably.[9,14,19,20]

MR enteroclysis provides better depiction of endoluminal lesions in the small intestine than that achieved on MR enterography,[21] especially at level of jejunal loops.[22] All sequences should be performed in breath-holds. The patient's position during imaging can be supine or prone. Prone positioning reduces the area to be imaged, and may help elevate small-bowel loops and separate them from the pelvis.[11,21] A preprocedural fasting time of 4 hours is recommended[23]; fasting reduces the amount of food residue and debris in the intestinal lumen, which may be mistaken for mass lesions or polyps. Most centers perform MR enterography with a torso coil at 1.5 T to enhance access and reproducibility of image quality. The pulse sequences used for both MR enteroclysis and MR enterography are essentially the same, the only difference being that breath-hold 2-dimensional T2-weighted fast spin-echo images are acquired continuously during the infusion of intraluminal contrast agent for MR enteroclysis, but only once for MR enterography.

Antiperistaltic agents are used to eliminate peristalsis and reduce motion artifact.[17] Achieving reduced peristalsis is of considerable importance for the T1-weighted 3-dimensional sequences performed after the administration of intravenous contrast material, and may help to limit intraluminal flow artifacts on images obtained with the half-Fourier acquisition.

The T2-weighted sequence based on the half-Fourier reconstruction technique, termed either half-Fourier RARE or single-shot fast spin-echo, allows each image to be obtained in less than 1 second, thereby overcoming or limiting artifacts arising from small-bowel peristalsis.[12] The coronal and axial balanced gradient-echo MR images that are obtained yield contrast that is intermediate relative to contrast on T1-weighted and T2-weighted images.

Balanced gradient-echo sequences (fast imaging employing steady-state acquisition [FIESTA] and true fast imaging with steady-state precession [TrueFISP]) are particularly effective as a means of obtaining information about mural and extraintestinal abnormalities.[24–26]

Coronal gradient-echo fat-saturated T1-weighted sequences are performed after gadolinium-based contrast material is administered (0.2 mmol per kilogram of body weight at a rate of 2 mL/s). The entire protocol for MR enterography takes 20 to 25 minutes, whereas 30 to 35 minutes are required for the MR enteroclysis protocol (excluding the time required for the fluoroscopically guided nasojejunal intubation), owing to the intraluminal administration of contrast medium through a nasojejunal catheter.

MR enteroclysis is a validated technique for the detection of small-bowel tumors and low-grade obstruction of small bowel, whereas MR enterography has not yet demonstrated its potential for these indications.[2,27,28] MR enteroclysis provides optimal small-bowel distension and allows more accurate detection of strictures.[18,21] Moreover, small polypoid masses that do not cause an obstruction may be difficult to detect using oral contrast material for distension.

IMAGE INTERPRETATION

The transit of the PEG solution through the small bowel is considered normal when unimpeded flow of intraluminal solution from the duodenojejunal junction to the ascending colon is observed, with no evidence of transit delay or stenosis during MR fluoroscopy.

Bowel-wall thickness of more than 3 mm must be considered abnormal.[1,29] MR imaging is able to assess the morphology of the lesion and the endoluminal, mural, and extramural abnormalities; these findings are relevant for the differential diagnosis of small-bowel neoplasms.

Small-bowel tumors are commonly mildly hypointense or isointense to the intestinal wall on precontrast T1-weighted sequences, show a variable grade of enhancement on postgadolinium images, and are better depicted with the use of fat-suppression techniques, which increase the conspicuity between the enhancing mass and the surrounding mesenteric fat.

The high signal intensity of the intraluminal fluid and mesenteric fat on TrueFISP and half-Fourier acquisition single-shot turbo spin-echo (HASTE) images allows the depiction of tumors exhibiting intermediate signal intensity.[29] High contrast between the tumors and surrounding bright fat enables MR imaging to accurately demonstrate the local extension of the lesions.[30]

BENIGN TUMORS
Adenoma

Adenomas are the most common benign and asymptomatic tumors of the small intestine, which occur frequently in the duodenum, in particular near the ampulla of Vater. Adenomas may have malignant potential, and the presence of numerous adenomas in the duodenum should lead one to consider familial adenomatous polyposis.

Adenomas have different types of growth, and may appear as polypoid pedunculated mass on a stalk, a sessile mass (broad-based and without a stalk), or a mural nodule within the mucosa. Adenomatous small-bowel polyps appear as intraluminal homogeneous enhancing masses on gadolinium-enhanced fat-suppressed images, confined within the boundaries of intestinal lumen.

On HASTE and TrueFISP sequences, polyps appear as rounded low–signal-intensity intraluminal masses (**Fig. 1**). MR fluoroscopy sequences show an intraluminal filling with no evidence of prestenotic dilatation.[29]

Polyposis Syndromes

Peutz-Jeghers syndrome is an autosomal dominant disease characterized by multiple hamartomatous polyps involving the small bowel, colon, and stomach, and mucocutaneous pigmentation involving the mouth, fingers, and toes.

Polyps have malignant potential and usually are asymptomatic, sometimes being determined by obstruction or bleeding.[31,32] Another common complication of Peutz-Jeghers syndrome is intussusception by a Peutz-Jeghers polyp. Although this concerns intussusceptions with a lead point, some of these resolve spontaneously.[31]

Because of the possible malignant evolution of polyps, surveillance of patients with Peutz-Jeghers syndrome has always been considered a major problem. International guidelines recommend biennial examination of the small bowel.[32] Conventional enteroclysis is no longer used

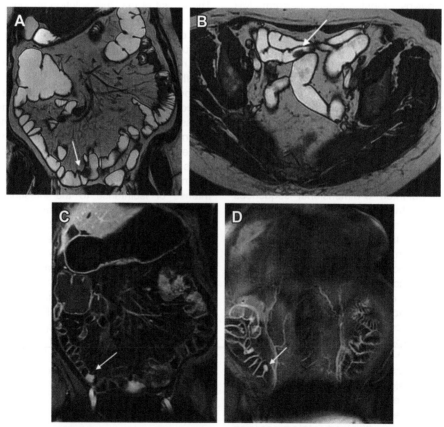

Fig. 1. MR enteroclysis images of a 73-year-old patient whit Peutz-Jeghers syndrome. Coronal (*A*) and axial (*B*) true fast imaging with steady-state precession (TrueFISP) images show a soft-tissue intraluminal mass (*arrow*), which appears moderately low in signal intensity, with no sign of bowel wall infiltration; note that the lesion is well circumscribed with lobulate borders and protrudes within the lumen of ileum distended by polyethylene glycol solution. (*C, D*) Coronal contrast T1-weighted fat-suppressed images show intense enhancement of the lesion (*arrow in C*) with evidence of another small polyp with a slender stalk (*arrow in D*).

because of the risk of cumulative radiation exposure associated with these tests.

Capsule endoscopy is probably the best method to visualize the mucosal abnormalities, and is usually the patient's preference.

MR enterography offers a promising alternative to capsule endoscopy for surveillance of patients with large polyps, given that it is more accurate in the estimation of location and size of the intraluminal abnormalities.[33,34]

No significant difference between MR enterography and wireless capsule endoscopy were found when used to detect large (>15 mm) clinically important polyps in patients with inherited polyposis syndromes, although MR imaging allowed more accurate localization of the polyps.[33–35] MR enterography may thus be used for routine surveillance in patients with large polyps alone, because small polyps are not clinically relevant.

In adults with Peutz-Jeghers syndrome, MR enterography may be less prone than capsule endoscopy to miss large polyps and may also provide more reliable size assessments of these polyps. In addition, MR enterography offers the potential for detecting extraluminal cancers in this patient group.

MR enterography performed by combining prone and supine position was accurate in the detection of Peutz-Jeghers syndrome polyps, with 93% concordance with enteroscopy for larger and more risky polyps.[35]

FISP and gadolinium-enhanced fat-suppressed volumetric interpolated breath-hold examination (VIBE) are the most useful MR imaging sequences for detecting small-bowel polyps. Polyps appear as hypointense filling defects on FISP images, and typically show marked enhancement similar to that of the bowel-wall mucosa after the intravenous administration of a gadolinium chelate.[29,32,33]

Lipoma

Lipomas are mature adipose tissue proliferations that arise in the submucosa of the bowel wall and frequently are seen in the distal small bowel. Lipomas are asymptomatic and are found incidentally, but when large they may produce ulceration and present iron-deficiency anemia or positive fecal occult blood testing.[36] These lesions usually grow intraluminally but can occasionally extend outward in the mesenteric surface, and the ileum is the most frequent location.[37]

Lipomas are high in signal intensity on T1-weighted images and have signal intensity comparable with that of intra-abdominal fat on T2-weighted images. On T1-weighted and T2-weighted fat-suppressed images these lesions show a loss of signal intensity, without enhancement on postgadolinium images.[2]

Hemangioma

Intestinal hemangiomas are congenital submucosal tumors, mostly located in the jejunum; they may consist of either capillaries or cavernous vessels, and most commonly manifest with acute or chronic bleeding of the GI tract. Hemangiomas can be sessile or pedunculated.[37]

Hemangiomas may appear as multiple nodules that show low signal intensity on T1-weighted images and marked hypersignal on T2-weighted images; central nodular enhancement is seen within the tumor in the arterial phase, with centrifugal enhancement on delayed phase. It may be difficult to differentiate hemangiomas from other vascular tumors or malformations based on imaging criteria alone.

Leiomyoma

Leiomyomas are mesenchymal tumors that do not express the c-KIT protein; they manifest themselves with nonspecific symptoms and bleeding. Leiomyomas are oval or round masses with a maximal diameter of 1 to 10 cm; they have intense uniform enhancement greater than that of adjacent bowel on postgadolinium images, reflecting similar imaging findings (**Fig. 2**).[38]

At MR fluoroscopy the leiomyoma appears as a smooth, round (or semilunar), mural defect that is demarcated by sharp angles to the intestinal wall. The typical findings and the absence of mesenteric changes and metastases helps in the diagnosis, and mostly rules out malignant differential diagnosis.

MALIGNANT TUMORS
Adenocarcinoma

Adenocarcinomas are malignant tumors of the glandular epithelium. These carcinomas represent 1% of all primary GI malignancies; they are the most common primary malignancy of the small bowel and occur in the majority of cases in the proximal intestine, duodenum, and jejunum.[36] Adenocarcinomas may be associated with Crohn disease, Peutz-Jeghers syndrome, and Lynch syndrome II, which represent risk factors for the onset of tumors.

Adenocarcinomas on MR imaging may appear as infiltrative lesions, causing luminal stenosis and obstruction with prestenotic dilatation, whereas polypoid intraluminal masses are less common. Ulceration is a common feature. Adenocarcinomas

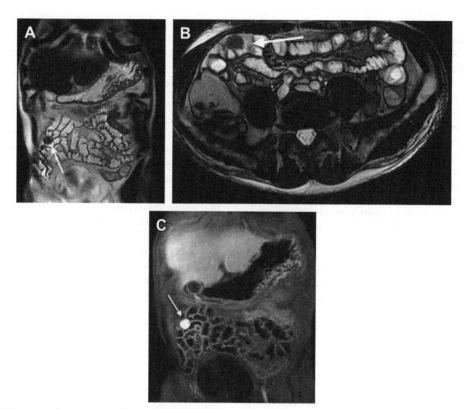

Fig. 2. MR enteroclysis images of a 63-year-old patient with ileal leiomyoma. Coronal half-Fourier acquisition single-shot turbo spin-echo (HASTE) (*A*) and axial (*B*) true fast imaging with steady-state precession (TrueFISP) sequences show a well-defined soft-tissue lesion, smoothly outlined (*arrow*), extending outside the intestinal wall of an ileal loop. (*C*) On axial contrast fat-saturated T1-weighted image, the lesion shows marked uniform enhancement after gadolinium (*arrow*).

tend to infiltrate the entire bowel wall and to extend into the surrounding mesenteric fat tissue.

Postgadolinium MR imaging typically demonstrates heterogeneous and moderate enhancement. MR fluoroscopy sequences show sharply demarcated, circumferential narrowing of the lumen, with shouldering of the margins and mucosal destruction (**Fig. 3**).[29]

Metastases from bowel adenocarcinomas to lymph nodes, liver, peritoneal surfaces, and ovaries may be depicted on MR enterography.[39–42]

The differential diagnosis is made possible by the demonstration of a solitary lesion, most frequently located proximally, which involves short segments of bowel and infiltrates perivisceral fat.

Gastrointestinal Stromal Tumor

Gastrointestinal stromal tumors (GISTs) constitute the major subset of GI mesenchymal neoplasms, encompassing most tumors previously classified as smooth-muscle tumors.[43–49]

GISTs comprise one-fifth of soft-tissue sarcomas, making them the most common single type of sarcoma.[49] The crude annual incidence of clinically detected GISTs is about 10 cases per million in Europe.[49,50] GISTs can arise at any age, although 80% occur in individuals older than 50 years.[49,51] About 0% to 4% of patients are younger than 20 years[49] and frequently have GIST associated with a syndrome.

GISTs occur anywhere along the GI tract: 50% to 60% in the stomach, 30% to 35% in the small intestine, and less frequently in the colon and rectum (5%) and esophagus (<1%).[49] This neoplasm, as opposed to smooth-muscle and neural tumors, express the KIT (CD117) protein, which allows it to be differentiated from other tumors. Most (70%–80%) of the tumors are benign, but 20% to 30% are malignant. Histopathologic predictors of malignancy are a size of more than 5 cm and a mitotic count of more than 5 mitoses per 50 high-powered fields.[52]

Small-bowel GISTs may produce various clinical manifestations, including melena from acute GI-tract bleeding secondary to mucosal ulceration, hematochezia, and hypovolemic shock. Chronic GI-tract bleeding may lead to anemia.

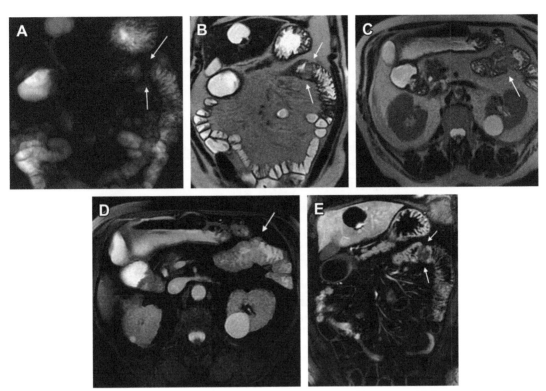

Fig. 3. MR enteroclysis image of jejunal adenocarcinoma in a 65-year-old patient with low-grade small-bowel obstruction. MR fluoroscopy image (*A*) shows mucosal irregularity, the typical annular lesion (*arrows*) suggesting malignant neoplasm originating from the mucosa at level of the proximal jejunum. Coronal (*B*) and axial (*C*) HASTE and Axial TrueFISP fat-saturated image (*D*) images show irregular short-segment circumferential thickening and stenosis. Contrast fat-saturated T1-weighted image (*E*) shows moderate enhancement of the lesion.

Small-bowel obstruction occurs rarely.[53] This type of tumor usually involves the muscular layer of the GI-tract wall; therefore, they have an exophytic growth pattern, but mucosa may be affected and ulcerations coexist in up to 50%.[43]

On MR imaging, different growth patterns are observed: GISTs may appear as a mass protruding in an intraluminal, extraluminal, or bidirectional fashion relative to the intestinal wall and lumen.[45] Malignant GISTs show slow growth, predominantly extraluminally and eccentrically, and frequently develop necrosis, hemorrhage, calcifications, fistula, or infection.

On MR imaging, tumors are typically of low signal intensity on T1-weighted images and high signal intensity on T2-weighted images, and enhance after administration of gadolinium. Areas of hemorrhage within the tumor will vary from high to low signal intensity on both T1-weighted and T2-weighted images, depending on the age of the hemorrhage. A homogeneous pattern of signal intensity is less common (**Fig. 4**).[54]

The differential diagnosis of GIST includes other mesenchymal tumors (leiomyomas, leiomyosarcomas, schwannomas), neuroendocrine tumors, primary carcinomas of the GI tract, lymphomas, or metastatic tumors, especially in the small bowel.[55]

Lymphoma

Lymphomas originate from lymphoid intestinal tissue (mucosa-associated lymphoid tissue) or may involve the bowel from widespread systemic disease. Non-Hodgkin B-cell lymphoma is the most common histologic subtype. Lymphomas represent about 20% of primary malignancies of the small intestine.[21,56] The ileum is the most common site of onset (due to the high amount of lymphoid tissue) while the duodenum is the least frequent site. Predisposing conditions are celiac disease, chronic lymphocytic leukemia, and immunoproliferative small-intestinal disease.[21]

Lymphomas may have different patterns of growth: (1) infiltrating lesions that may produce full-thickness mural with effacement of overlying

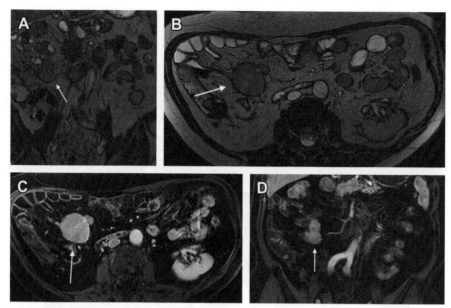

Fig. 4. MR enteroclysis images of jejunal gastrointestinal stromal in a 77-year-old man with unexplained gastrointestinal bleeding. Coronal (*A*) and axial (*B*) TrueFISP images show lobulated mass that arises from a jejunal loop, with smooth borders and extraluminal growth (*arrow*); Axial (*C*) and coronal (*D*) contrast T1-weighted LAVA sequences show heterogeneous intense enhancement.

mucosal folds; (2) polypoid lesions that protrude into the lumen; and (3) large, exophytic, fungating masses that are prone to ulceration and fistula formation (**Figs. 5** and **6**). Another characteristic of the growth of lymphomas is aneurysmal dilatation of the lumen, caused by the loss of tone of intestinal musculature invaded and destroyed by pathologic tissue.[21,56] On MR fluoroscopic sequences, an infiltrative lesion with patency of bowel lumen or a nonstenotic bowel mass is suggestive of lymphoma. The presence of mesenteric involvement with enlarged lymph nodes is another feature. Splenomegaly and mesenteric and retroperitoneal lymphadenopathy support the diagnosis.[21]

Smooth mural contour, diffuse or segmental bowel-loop aneurysmal dilatation, and absence of a distinct mesenteric or antimesenteric distribution are highly suggestive of the presence of lymphoma in patients with celiac disease.[12,21,57] Thickening of the small-bowel wall and luminal stenosis are found in both neoplastic and inflammatory diseases.

An adenocarcinoma may be easily confused with a lymphoma, but the former, in addition to mesenteric fat infiltration, presents lymph node metastases as much more bulky.

The differential diagnosis must be made with respect to inflammatory small-bowel diseases such as intestinal tuberculosis and infectious diseases, conditions characterized by thickened small-bowel wall and luminal stenosis; also present are edema, ulcerations, increased mesenteric

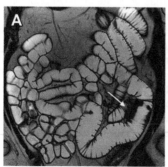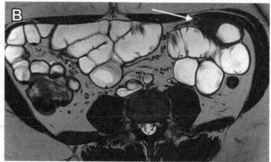

Fig. 5. MR enteroclysis images of jejunal lymphoma in a 32-year-old man with unexplained gastrointestinal bleeding. Coronal (*A*) and axial (*B*) TrueFISP images show a segment of jejunum (*arrow*) with abnormal wall thickening, smooth margins, and loss of normal mucosal folds.

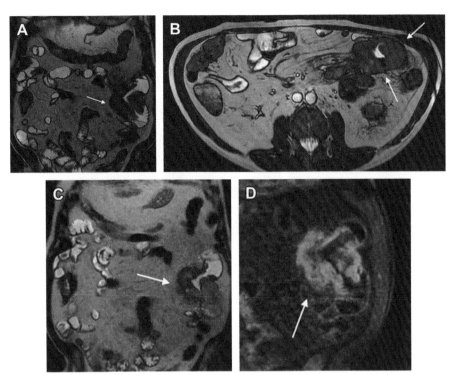

Fig. 6. MR enterography images of a 73-year-old man with follicular B-cell non-Hodgkin jejunal lymphoma. Coronal (*A*) and axial (*B*) TrueFISP images show a mass (*arrows*) infiltrating the jejunal small bowel, which appears dilated. Coronal HASTE sequence (*C*) shows a segment of jejunum (*arrow*) with abnormal thickening, smooth margins, and luminal narrowing with loss of normal mucosal folds. Coronal contrast T1-weighted LAVA sequence (*D*) shows minimal enhancement of the mass (*arrow*) infiltrating the small-bowel loop.

vascularization (comb sign), enhancing mesenteric lymph nodes, and increased mesenteric fat. In acute inflammation, the bowel wall can have a layered pattern resulting from submucosal edema, which is not seen in neoplastic diseases.

Intestinal Neuroendocrine Tumor

Carcinoids are well-differentiated endocrine tumors that arise from the enterochromograffin cells at the base of the crypts of Lieberkuhn, accounting for nearly 25% of primary malignant small-bowel neoplasms.[28] Carcinoid tumors cause focal, asymmetric bowel-wall thickening and usually manifest as nodular wall thickening or a smooth submucosal mass.

The most common sites of occurrence are the appendix (50%) and the distal ileum. Symptoms are often nonspecific, and because the tumor has very slow growth it may go unrecognized for many years.

Tumors secreting serotonin usually induce a typical sclerosis and retraction of the adjacent mesenteric stroma, thus producing a sharp bend in the lumen. Only 10% of patients develop carcinoid syndrome[58] attributable to serotonin secreted by the tumors.

MR fluoroscopy shows solitary or multiple round, intramural, or intraluminal filling defects encroaching on the intestinal lumen.

Carcinoid neoplasm causes kinking of the bowel wall, with secondary narrowing of the lumen, rather than annular stenosis.[2,28] These lesions are isointense to muscle on T1-weighted images and isointense or mildly hyperintense to muscle on T2-weighted images. The primary lesions show contrast enhancement. Mesenteric masses range between 2 and 4 cm and are typically isointense to muscle on T1-weighted and T2-weighted images (**Fig. 7**).

Hypervascular metastases may be seen in the liver[59]; enlarged lymph nodes and ascites caused by peritoneal seeding are also possible.

Leiomyosarcoma

Leiomyosarcomas arise from the wall of smooth muscle or from small blood vessels. Usually leiomyosarcomas grow slowly, extraluminally and eccentrically, to a size exceeding 5 cm.

On MR imaging, leiomyosarcomas appear as large heterogeneous masses, with central necrosis and hemorrhage. MR fluoroscopy shows a

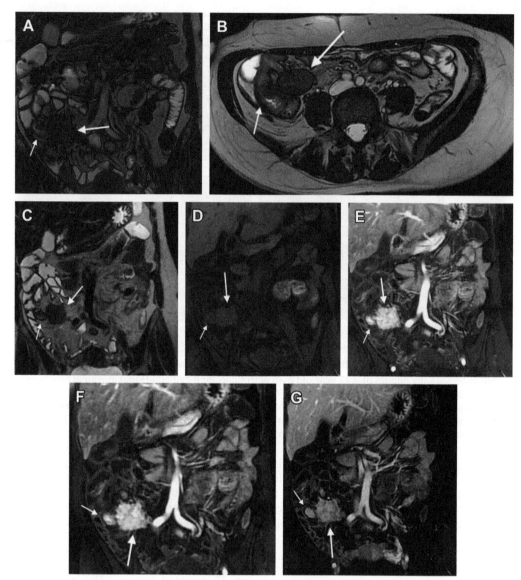

Fig. 7. MR enteroclysis images of ileal carcinoid neoplasm in a 59-year-old woman with unexplained gastrointestinal bleeding. Coronal (*A*) and axial (*B*) TrueFISP and coronal HASTE (*C*) images show spiculated mesenteric mass (*arrow*) with desmoplastic reaction and a small intraluminal lesion at the level of terminal ileum (*short arrow*). The masses are better depicted on coronal contrast-enhanced T1-weighted volumetric interpolated breath-hold examination (VIBE) images (*D–G*), which show a small hypervascular nodule (*short arrow*) in the lumen of the small bowel (the primary tumor).

large extrinsic mass, displacing or distorting adjacent loops.

The differential diagnosis is made from leiomyoma, but this usually is smaller and does not show areas of necrosis or heterogeneous tissue intensity.[28]

Celiac Disease

The pathologic changes of celiac disease are predominantly seen in the duodenum and proximal jejunum. However, the extent of the disease is extremely variable, ranging from segmental to full involvement of the small bowel.[57] The most specific sign of celiac disease is fold-pattern abnormalities.[2] Abnormalities of the intestinal fold pattern are defined qualitatively as a decreased number of jejunal folds.

Valvulae conniventes may exhibit different patterns: (1) normal: in most patients valvulae look normal; (2) squared ends: ends at the margin are squared off rather than rounded; (3) reversed jejunal fold pattern: decreased jejunal folds with increased ileal folds; and (4) absence of valvulae: Moulage sign, characteristic of sprue, caused by total villous atrophy The small-bowel findings in celiac disease reflect the underlying villous atrophy. With extensive villous atrophy, there is loss of the surface area of the mucosa. This loss of mucosa in celiac disease is manifested by a decreased number of folds in the proximal jejunum, the portion of the small bowel most severely involved in the disease.

Jejunal folds should be considered decreased in number if there are fewer than 3 folds per inch. In severe celiac disease a complete flattening of jejunal folds can be observed. An increased number of ileal folds (>5 per inch) represents another specific sign of celiac disease (**Fig. 8**).

A reversed jejunoileal fold pattern, which presumably is caused by a compensatory response of the ileum to severe villous atrophy of the proximal small bowel, is highly suggestive of celiac disease. Small-bowel dilatation, affecting particularly the jejunum, is commonly found in celiac patients and is believed to occur secondarily to intestinal hypomobility.

Alteration of bowel-wall thickness represents an uncommon and nonspecific sign of celiac disease. Mural thickening in the setting of celiac disease may reflect submucosal edema and varying degrees of inflammation.

Bowel wall is considered thickened when it measures more than 4 mm. Bowel-wall thickening is usually diffuse and is not associated with reduction of intestinal caliber. Intestinal strictures are not common in celiac disease, and do not represent a specific sign of disease.

Benign mesenteric lymphadenopathies are the most common extraintestinal findings (reported in up to 42% of the patients), and usually are caused by reactive lymphoid hyperplasia. Mesenteric vascular engorgement is defined as increased caliber of both mesenteric arteries and veins. Although it is a common finding in celiac disease, it does not represent a specific sign of celiac disease.

The T2-weighted single-shot echo-train technique may demonstrate an abnormal mucosal fold pattern of the small bowel, associated with an increase of intraluminal fluid.[57] Endoscopic biopsy is required for a definitive diagnosis of celiac

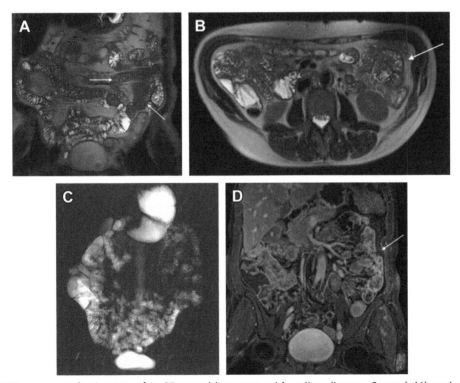

Fig. 8. MR enterography images of a 35-year-old woman with celiac disease. Coronal (*A*) and axial (*B*) T2-weighted HASTE images of a patient with celiac disease show smooth thickening of jejunal ileal loops (*arrows*). MR fluoroscopy sequence (*C*) in the same patient shows increased number of folds along ileal loops. Coronal contrast T1-weighted LAVA (*D*) shows homogeneous enhancement of the jejunal and ileal small-bowel wall, with absence of bowel thickening (*arrow*).

disease, although MR studies may also be performed to establish the diagnosis in patients with atypical symptoms.

MR imaging modalities can provide morphologic information obtained noninvasively, such as fold-pattern abnormalities and bowel dilatation, as well as extraintestinal findings, such as mesenteric vascular congestion, lymphadenopathy, hyposplenism, and the presence of intussusceptions.

COMPARISON WITH OTHER MODALITIES

MR enteroclysis has yielded a 96.6% accuracy in the detection of small-bowel neoplasms, thereby proving to be an effective means of diagnosing or ruling out small-bowel neoplasms[2,10]; interobserver MR enteroclysis agreement is also excellent.[2] By contrast, MR enterography has not yet displayed the same potential.[34]

MR enteroclysis has proved to be more sensitive than computed tomography (CT) enteroclysis for detecting mucosal lesions of the small bowel,[38] and it appears to facilitate superior detection of segments with only superficial abnormalities. These findings may be due to the better soft-tissue contrast afforded by MR imaging, which is required for tissue characterization and the detection of subtle areas of abnormality,[10,60] and its functional capabilities. An intermittent spasm or peristaltic contraction during a CT examination may instead be misdiagnosed as a small-bowel neoplasm.[19] Another advantage of MR imaging over CT is that the former technique provides more information regarding the nature of the mesenteric small-bowel tumor, thereby providing a higher degree of small-bowel tumor characterization.[34]

In this regard, benign tumors such as hemangiomas are typically strongly hyperintense on T2-weighted MR imaging, whereas lipomas or tumors with a marked fat content are spontaneously hyperintense on T1-weighted MR images.[34,60] Fat content can be confirmed by a combination of sequences that are pathognomonic for fat.

In addition, the findings yielded by MR enteroclysis can be used to differentiate between benign and malignant neoplasms.[2] Small-bowel tumors usually exhibit moderate signal intensity on True-FISP images, in contrast to the high signal intensity of the distended lumen and mesenteric fat.

Imaging features associated with small-bowel malignancy are the presence of longer solitary nonpedunculated lesions, mesenteric fat infiltration, and enlarged mesenteric lymph nodes.[2,10]

The MR signal appearance of intraluminal, mural, and mesenteric neoplastic manifestations can help in the differential diagnosis of small-bowel neoplasms.[10,34]

Small-bowel wall thickness and luminal stenosis can be seen in both neoplastic and inflammatory diseases. In acute inflammation, the bowel wall may have a layered pattern on contrast-enhanced T1-weighted images and high signal intensity on fat-saturated T2-weighted images because of submucosal edema, which is not seen in neoplastic diseases.[9] Moreover, inflammatory stenoses are usually located at the terminal ileum, which are multiple and longer than neoplastic stenoses.[10]

Dynamic cine MR sequences can be used to assess the distensibility of the stenoses, which varies in inflammatory conditions but remains unchanged in neoplastic disease.

Lymphoma can, in some cases, mimic inflammatory bowel disease; the homogeneous signal on T2-weighted sequences combined with lymph node enlargement and splenomegaly allows it to be differentiated from Crohn disease.[9]

The use of capsule endoscopy to evaluate small-bowel tumors, particularly submucosal forms, has several limitations.[61,62] One such limitation is the difficulty encountered in identifying the abnormality and tumor type based on the capsule endoscopic appearance of the lesions. Indeed, capsule endoscopy may fail to detect neoplastic disease in as many as 18.9% of cases.[63]

Another major limitation of wireless capsule endoscopy is capsule retention in 10% to 25% of cases of small-bowel tumor,[61,64] which thus restricts its use in patients with suspected small-bowel neoplasms.

MR enteroclysis may be considered the modality of choice because of its accuracy in the diagnosis of small-bowel neoplasms. In patients with obscure gastrointestinal bleeding, MR enteroclysis may be used to accurately detect inflammatory and neoplastic diseases, as well as other conditions that cause bleeding, such as Meckel diverticulum. Therefore, when MR enteroclysis is negative and an arteriovenous malformation is likely to be the cause of bleeding, endoscopy may be required for the diagnosis and treatment of such malformations. The authors thus believe that MR enteroclysis should precede enteroscopic modalities in the examination of patients with obscure GI bleeding.[27]

SUMMARY

MR imaging can provide exquisite anatomic, functional, and real-time information without the need for ionizing radiation in the evaluation of small-bowel tumors.

MR enteroclysis may be considered the best radiologic modality for the examination of the small bowel, and should be recommended for the initial investigation in patients suspected of having small-bowel tumors.[7,65] MR-signal appearances of the lesions, combined with the contrast-enhancement behavior and the characteristics of the stenosis, can help in differentiating from other nonneoplastic diseases of the small bowel.[57,66–68]

Furthermore, MR imaging may be used for follow-up and detection of the complications of celiac disease, such as those observed in celiac disease complicated by small-bowel malignancy.

REFERENCES

1. Fork FT, Aabakken L. Capsule enteroscopy and radiology of the small intestine. Eur Radiol 2007; 17:3103–11.
2. Van Weyenberg SJ, Meijerink MR, Jacobs MA, et al. MR enteroclysis in the diagnosis of small bowel neoplasms. Radiology 2010;254:765–73.
3. Rieber A, Aschoff A, Nüssle K, et al. MRI in the diagnosis of small bowel disease: use of positive and negative oral contrast media in combination with enteroclysis. Eur Radiol 2000;10(9):1377–82.
4. Small WC, DeSimone-Macchi D, Parker JR, et al. A multisite phase III study of the safety and efficacy of a new manganese chloride-based gastrointestinal contrast agent for MRI of the abdomen and pelvis. J Magn Reson Imaging 1999;10(1):15–24.
5. Kivelitz D, Gehl HB, Heuck A, et al. Ferric ammonium citrate as a positive bowel contrast agent for MR imaging of the upper abdomen. Safety and diagnostic efficacy. Acta Radiol 1999;40(4): 429–35.
6. Karantanas AH, Papanikolaou N, Kalef-Ezra J, et al. Blueberry juice used per os in upper abdominal MR imaging: composition and initial clinical data. Eur Radiol 2000;10(6):909–13.
7. Schreyer AG, Gölder S, Scheibl K, et al. Dark lumen magnetic resonance enteroclysis in combination with MRI colonography for whole bowel assessment in patients with Crohn's disease: first clinical experience. Inflamm Bowel Dis 2005; 11(4):388–94.
8. Gore R, Masselli G, Caroline D. Crohn's disease of the small bowel. In: Gore R, Levine M, editors. Textbook of gastrointestinal radiology. 3rd edition. Philadelphia: Saunders Elsevier; 2008. p. 781–806.
9. Umschaden HW, Gasser J. MR enteroclysis. Radiol Clin North Am 2003;41(2):231–48.
10. Masselli G, Polettini E, Casciani E, et al. Small-bowel neoplasms: prospective evaluation of MR enteroclysis. Radiology 2009;251(3):743–50.
11. Gourtsoyiannis N, Papanikolaou N, Grammatikakis J, et al. MR enteroclysis: technical considerations and clinical applications. Eur Radiol 2002;12(11):2651–8.
12. Masselli G, Picarelli A, Di Tola M, et al. Celiac disease: evaluation with dynamic contrast-enhanced MR imaging. Radiology 2010;256(3):783–90.
13. Low RN, Chen SC, Barone R. Distinguishing benign from malignant bowel obstruction in patients with malignancy: findings at MR imaging. Radiology 2003;228(1):157–65.
14. Gourtsoyiannis NC, Papanikolaou N. Magnetic resonance enteroclysis. Semin Ultrasound CT MR 2005;26(4):237–46.
15. Masselli G, Casciani E, Polettini E, et al. Assessment of Crohn's disease in the small bowel: prospective comparison of magnetic resonance enteroclysis with conventional enteroclysis. Eur Radiol 2006;16(12):2817–27.
16. Cronin CG, Lohan DG, Browne AM, et al. Magnetic resonance enterography in the evaluation of the small bowel. Semin Roentgenol 2009;44(4):237–43.
17. Umschaden HW, Szolar D, Gasser J, et al. Small-bowel disease: comparison of MR enteroclysis images with conventional enteroclysis and surgical findings. Radiology 2000;215(3):717–25.
18. Masselli G, Brizi MG, Menchini L, et al. Magnetic resonance enteroclysis of Crohn's. Radiol Med 2005;110:221–33.
19. Maglinte DD, Sandrasegaran K, Chiorean M, et al. Radiologic investigations complement and add diagnostic information to capsule endoscopy of small-bowel diseases. AJR Am J Roentgenol 2007;189(2):306–12.
20. Kelvin FM, Maglinte DD. Enteroclysis or small bowel follow-through in Crohn's diseases? Gastroenterology 1998;114(6):1349–51.
21. Masselli G, Casciani E, Polettini E, et al. Comparison of MR enteroclysis with MR enterography and conventional enteroclysis in patients with Crohn's disease. Eur Radiol 2008;18(3):438–47.
22. Negaard A, Paulsen V, Sandvik L, et al. A prospective randomized comparison between two MRI studies of the small bowel in Crohn's disease, the oral contrast method and MR enteroclysis. Eur Radiol 2007;17:2294–301.
23. Lin MF, Narra V. Developing role of magnetic resonance imaging in Crohn's disease. Curr Opin Gastroenterol 2008;24(2):135–40.
24. Prassopoulos P, Papanikolaou N, Grammatikakis J, et al. MR enteroclysis imaging of Crohn disease. Radiographics 2001;21:S161–72.
25. Wiarda BM, Horsthuis K, Dobben AC, et al. Magnetic resonance imaging of the small bowel with the true FISP sequence: intra- and interobserver agreement of enteroclysis and imaging without contrast material. Clin Imaging 2009;33(4):267–73.
26. Leyendecker JR, Bloomfeld RS, DiSantis DJ, et al. MR enterography in the management of patients with Crohn disease. Radiographics 2009;29(6): 1827–46.

27. Masselli G, Gualdi G. MR imaging of the small bowel. Radiology 2012;264(2):333–48.

28. Gourtsoyiannis N, Ji H, Odze RD. Malignant small intestinal neoplasm. In: Baert AL, Sartor K, editors. Radiological imaging of the small intestine. Berlin: Springer-Verlag; 2002. p. 399–428.

29. Masselli G, Gualdi G. Evaluation of small bowel tumors: MR enteroclysis. Abdom Imaging 2010;35:23–30.

30. Fidler JL, Guimaraes L, Einstein DM. MR imaging of the small bowel. Radiographics 2009;29:1811–25.

31. Rufener SL, Koujok K, McKenna BJ, et al. Small bowel intussusception secondary to Peutz-Jeghers polyp. Radiographics 2008;28:284–8.

32. Kopacova M, Tacheci I, Rejchrt S, et al. Peutz-Jeghers syndrome: diagnostic and therapeutic approach. World J Gastroenterol 2009;15:5397–408.

33. Gupta A, Postgate AJ, Burling D, et al. A prospective study of MR enterography versus capsule endoscopy for the surveillance of adult patients with Peutz-Jeghers syndrome. AJR Am J Roentgenol 2010;195(1):108–16.

34. Maccioni F, Al Ansari N, Mazzamurro F, et al. Surveillance of patients affected by Peutz-Jeghers syndrome: diagnostic value of MR enterography in prone and supine position. Abdom Imaging 2012;37(2):279–87.

35. Caspari R, von Falkenhausen M, Krautmacher C, et al. Comparison of capsule endoscopy and magnetic resonance imaging for the detection of polyps of the small intestine in patients with familial adenomatous polyposis or with Peutz-Jeghers' syndrome. Endoscopy 2004;36(12):1054–9.

36. Taylor AJ, Stewart ET, Dodds WJ. Gastrointestinal lipomas: a radiologic and pathologic review. AJR Am J Roentgenol 1990;155(6):1205–10.

37. Maglinte DD, Lappas JC, Sandrasegaran K. Malignant tumors of the small bowel. In: Gore R, Levine M, editors. Textbook of gastrointestinal radiology. 3rd edition. Philadelphia: Saunders Elsevier; 2008. p. 853–69.

38. Semelka RC, John G, Kalekis N, et al. Small bowel neoplastic disease: demonstration by MRI. J Magn Reson Imaging 1996;6:855–60.

39. Madani G, Katz RD, Haddock JA, et al. The role of radiology in the management of systemic sclerosis. Clin Radiol 2008;63(9):959–67.

40. Ramachandran I, Sinha R, Rajesh A, et al. Multidetector row CT of small bowel tumours. Clin Radiol 2007;62(7):607–14.

41. Hyland R, Chalmers A. CT features of jejunal pathology. Clin Radiol 2007;62(12):1154–62.

42. Wiarda BM, Heine DG, Rombouts MC, et al. Jejunum abnormalities at MR enteroclysis. Eur J Radiol 2008;67(1):125–32.

43. Levy AD, Remotti HE, Thompson WM, et al. Gastrointestinal stromal tumors: radiologic features with pathologic correlation. Radiographics 2003;23:283–304.

44. Burkill GJ, Badran M, Al-Muderis O, et al. Malignant gastrointestinal stromal tumor: distribution, imaging features, and pattern of metastatic spread. Radiology 2003;226:527–32.

45. Lappas JC, Maglinte DD, Sandrasegaran K. Benign tumors of the small bowel. In: Gore R, Levine M, editors. Textbook of gastrointestinal radiology. 3rd edition. Philadelphia: Saunders Elsevier; 2008. p. 845–51.

46. Agaimy A. Gastrointestinal stromal tumors (GIST) from risk stratification systems to the new TNM proposal: more questions than answers? A review emphasizing the need for a standardized GIST reporting. Int J Clin Exp Pathol 2010;3:461–71.

47. Strickland L, Letson GD, Muro-Cacho CA. Gastrointestinal stromal tumors. Cancer Control 2001;8:252–61.

48. Fletcher CD, Berman JJ, Corless C, et al. Diagnosis of gastrointestinal stromal tumors: a consensus approach. Hum Pathol 2002;33:459–65.

49. Ducimetière F, Lurkin A, Ranchère-Vince D, et al. Incidence of sarcoma histotypes and molecular subtypes in a prospective epidemiological study with central pathology review and molecular testing. PLoS One 2011;6:e20294.

50. Nilsson B, Bümming P, Meis-Kindblom JM, et al. Gastrointestinal stromal tumors: the incidence, prevalence, clinical course, and prognostication in the preimatinib mesylate era—a population-based study in western Sweden. Cancer 2005;103:821–9.

51. Joensuu H, Vehtari A, Riihimäki J, et al. Risk of recurrence of gastrointestinal stromal tumour after surgery: an analysis of pooled population-based cohorts. Lancet Oncol 2012;13:265–74.

52. Emory TS, Sobin LH, Lukes L, et al. Prognosis of gastrointestinal smooth-muscle (stromal) tumors: dependence on anatomic site. Am J Surg Pathol 1999;23(1):82–7.

53. Amzallag-Bellenger E, Oudjit A, Ruiz A, et al. Effectiveness of MR enterography for the assessment of small-bowel diseases beyond Crohn disease. Radiographics 2012;32(5):1423–44.

54. Masselli G, Colaiacomo MC, Marcelli G, et al. MRI of the small-bowel: how to differentiate primary neoplasms and mimickers. Br J Radiol 2012;85(1014):824–37.

55. Kavaliauskiene G, Ziech ML, Nio CY, et al. Small bowel MRI in adult patients: not just Crohn's disease—a tutorial. Insights Imaging 2011;2(5):501–13.

56. Ghai S, Pattison J, Ghai S, et al. Primary gastrointestinal lymphoma: spectrum of imaging findings and pathologic correlation. Radiographics 2007;27:1371–88.

57. Di Sabatino A, Corazza GR. Coeliac disease. Lancet 2009;373(9673):1480–93.

58. Horton KM, Kamel I, Hofmann L, et al. Carcinoid tumors of the small bowel: a multitechnique imaging approach. AJR Am J Roentgenol 2004;182(3): 559–67.

59. Hoeffel C, Crema MD, Belkacem A, et al. Multidetector row CT: spectrum of diseases involving the ileocecal area. Radiographics 2006;26(5): 1373–90.

60. Albert JG, Martiny F, Krummenerl A, et al. Diagnosis of small bowel Crohn's disease: a prospective comparison of capsule endoscopy with magnetic resonance imaging and fluoroscopic enteroclysis. Gut 2005;54(12):1721–7.

61. Postgate A, Despott E, Burling D, et al. Significant small-bowel lesions detected by alternative diagnostic modalities after negative capsule endoscopy. Gastrointest Endosc 2008;68(6): 1209–14.

62. Baichi MM, Arifuddin RM, Mantry PS. Small-bowel masses found and missed on capsule endoscopy for obscure bleeding. Scand J Gastroenterol 2007;42(9):1127–32.

63. Pennazio M, Rondonotti E, de Franchis R. Capsule endoscopy in neoplastic diseases. World J Gastroenterol 2008;14(34):5245–53.

64. Estévez E, González-Conde B, Vázquez-Iglesias JL, et al. Incidence of tumoral pathology according to study using capsule endoscopy for patients with obscure gastrointestinal bleeding. Surg Endosc 2007;21(10):1776–80.

65. Green PH, Cellier C. Celiac disease. N Engl J Med 2007;357(17):1731–43.

66. Masselli G, Picarelli A, Gualdi G. Celiac disease: MR enterography and contrast enhanced MRI. Abdom Imaging 2010;35(4):399–406.

67. Masselli G, Gualdi G. CT and MR enterography in evaluating small bowel diseases: when to use which modality? Abdom Imaging 2013;38(2): 249–59.

68. Masselli G, Casciani E, Polettini E, et al. Magnetic resonance imaging of small bowel neoplasms. Cancer Imaging 2013;13:92–9.

Magnetic Resonance Colonography for Screening and Diagnosis of Colorectal Cancer

Marije P. van der Paardt, MD*, Jaap Stoker, MD, PhD

KEYWORDS

- Magnetic resonance imaging • Colonography • MR colonography • Screening • Colon • Neoplasm
- Polyps • Colorectal cancer

KEY POINTS

- Magnetic resonance (MR) colonography is a potential technique for colorectal cancer screening because of its lack of ionizing radiation and high soft-tissue contrast, thus rendering exceptional extracolonic assessment.
- Prerequisites of MR colonography are a bowel preparation with fecal tagging and adequate colonic distension.
- The results of diagnostic performance of MR colonography are promising but heterogeneous, which hampers the use of this modality as a screening tool for colorectal cancer at present.

INTRODUCTION

Colorectal cancer is the second most common cause of cancer-related death in Europe and the United States,[1,2] and is a major cause of mortality.[3] In 2012, an estimated 143,460 new cases were diagnosed with colorectal cancer in the United States.[3] The 5-year relative survival rate is 90.1%, if colorectal cancers are detected at a localized stage. However, when it has spread to regional lymph nodes and organs, the 5-year survival decreases to 69.2% and when it has metastasized to other than regional areas, survival decreases even further to 11.7%.[3] Early detection of colorectal cancer is therefore essential for high survival rates. Moreover, colorectal cancer can be prevented, as precancerous adenomatous polyps can be detected and removed. It is estimated that screening for colorectal cancer can reduce colorectal mortality by more than 50%.[4]

Different screening tools such as fecal occult blood tests (FOBT), barium contrast enema, sigmoidoscopy, and colonoscopy have been evaluated. Among these procedures, optical colonoscopy is the most accurate means for examining the colon, with high sensitivity and specificity regarding the detection of colorectal cancer and adenomatous polyps, with polypectomy reducing mortality rates of colorectal cancer.[2,4] Nevertheless, moderate patient acceptance has been demonstrated for screening programs in comparison with other screening methods (ie, FOBT), the participation rate of colonoscopy is demonstrably lower (FOBT 47%, colonoscopy 22%).[5]

The authors have nothing to disclose.

Department of Radiology, Academic Medical Center, University of Amsterdam, Meibergdreef 9, Amsterdam 1105 AZ, The Netherlands

* Corresponding author.

E-mail address: m.p.vanderpaardt@amc.uva.nl

In the 1990s the first attempts were made to develop an imaging-based minimally invasive technique for the detection of colorectal cancer and its precursors.[6,7] The available structural examinations (ie, optical colonoscopy and sigmoidoscopy), were subject to patient discomfort,[8] which led to the development of both computed tomography (CT) colonography and MR colonography. CT colonography was described first, and initial attempts were challenging because of time-consuming image reconstructions, disk-storage capacities, and the development of patient-preparation methods to avoid false-positive and false-negative findings.[6] Since then tremendous progress has been made in spatial resolution and the examination and interpretation times of CT colonography, and it is nowadays part of daily clinical practice.[9,10] Moreover, CT colonography has proved to be highly accurate in detecting colorectal cancer and large lesions of 10 mm and greater. In both average-risk and high-risk individuals, detection of precursors of colorectal carcinoma is high: per-patient sensitivity is 88% for advanced neoplasia of 10 mm or larger in screening populations and 96% for colorectal carcinoma in average-risk and high-risk populations, findings comparable with those of colonoscopy.[11,12] This success has resulted in the recommendation of CT colonography as a screening tool for colorectal cancer by the American Cancer Society.[2]

The major advantage over colonoscopy and sigmoidoscopy is that colonography (also known as virtual colonoscopy) lacks the need of sedation and a cathartic bowel preparation. Moreover, the risk of procedural complications is lower.[13]

Substantially more data are available on the diagnostic performance of CT colonography in comparison with MR colonography. CT colonography has the advantage of shorter examination times, clinical availability, and lower costs.[14] However, the major motivation to use MR colonography is the lack of ionizing radiation. This issue seems to be of lesser importance as the daily dose of radiation with CT colonography has been significantly reduced.[15] Nonetheless, evaluation of the complete colon without the use of ionizing radiation would be most favorable, as ionizing radiation might be a concern when used for screening purposes.[16] This aspect is especially important because screening by colonography most likely will not be limited to a single examination. Moreover, the excellent soft-tissue contrast of MR imaging has made MR colonography attractive for the evaluation of other abdominal abnormality (eg, inflammatory bowel disease, which is

described in an article elsewhere in this issue by Jordi and colleagues).

The aim of this review is to describe the current status and potential for MR colonography in screening for colorectal cancer.

NORMAL ANATOMY

For evaluation of the colon with colonography, the colon is divided into 6 colon segments: cecum, ascending colon, transverse colon, descending colon, sigmoid, and rectum (**Fig. 1**). For colorectal screening purposes, the colon is further divided into right colon, consisting of cecum, ascending colon, and transverse colon, and left colon, consisting of descending colon, sigmoid, and rectum. The location of the colon segments is either intraperitoneal or retroperitoneal. The cecum, transverse colon, and sigmoid colon lie intraperitoneal, whereas the other colon segments are retroperitoneal and are therefore fixed to the surroundings. This situation has an impact on the surgical approach to removal of colon tumors but also on the evaluation of the colon segments in dual positioning (see the section on imaging technique), as the intraperitoneal segments especially may displace. The colonic segments are collapsed or slightly distended by stool under normal physiologic circumstances. For evaluation with colonography, distension is essential (see later discussion).

PATHOLOGY

Colorectal cancer arises from adenomas presenting as luminal polyps, which are defined as

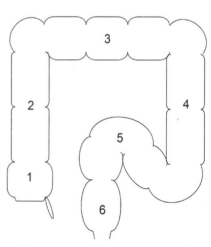

Fig. 1. Colon segments. 1, cecum; 2, ascending colon; 3, transverse colon; 4, descending colon; 5, sigmoid; 6, rectum.

protuberance of colonic-wall mucosa.[17] Screening for colorectal cancer should therefore not only focus on mass lesion detection suspected for colorectal carcinoma, but should also focus on its precursors to prevent progression to colorectal carcinoma.

Polyps have different morphologic features. Sessile polyps protrude more than 3 mm into the lumen.[18] A pedunculated polyp consists of a fine stalk attached to the mucosa. Different definitions are used for flat polyps, but in general the protrusion into the lumen should not be more than 3 mm for a polyp larger or equal to 6 mm in diameter.[18,19] Morphology is important in matching a lesion to colonoscopy results.

Development of colorectal cancer from colorectal polyps is related to both size and histology.[17] In general, polyps are categorized in diminutive (<6 mm), intermediate (6–9 mm), and large (≥10 mm) polyps.[17] Diminutive polyps harbor a low risk of advanced abnormality (0.5%) and intermediate polyps a higher risk (1.5%), whereas in polyps of 10 mm and larger the risk of advanced disease is 15% overall.[20]

Histology is a different prognostic factor for polyp progression to colorectal cancer. Most polyps are represented by hyperplastic polyps and adenomas. Adenomas are considered precursors of colorectal cancer, as they start as small lesions that progress to larger adenomas with dysplasia, and finally progress to invasive colorectal carcinoma.[21] Furthermore, small adenomas showing high-grade dysplasia and a villous component of greater than 25% are at high risk for development of colorectal cancer. Therefore, adenomas of 10 mm and larger, or with high-grade dysplasia or a villous component, are defined as advanced adenomas. Advanced adenomas and colorectal carcinomas are further defined as advanced neoplasia. These groups are of special interest to screening for colorectal cancer.

Recently a subset of both hyperplastic polyps and adenomas, known as sessile serrated adenomas, was shown to have different molecular alterations and also a high risk of malignancy. However, there is limited available evidence on the clinical implications for follow-up of patients with sessile serrated adenomas.[21,22]

Colonography cannot histologically differentiate detected polyps. Nevertheless, for screening purposes the detection rates of advanced adenomas and advanced neoplasias are relevant performance categories. For CT colonography the largest diameter of lesions should be estimated, and lesions of 6 mm and larger should be reported.[18] For MR colonography such consensus does not exist at the moment, but a similar approach seems sensible.

IMAGING TECHNIQUE

Colonic assessment with MR colonography requires bowel preparation and distension of the colon (**Box 1**). In MR colonography, the bright and dark-lumen strategy refers to the signal intensity of the bowel lumen at T1-weighted imaging.[23] In bright-lumen colonography, the bowel lumen is of high signal intensity and the colonic wall remains low in signal intensity. Detection of colonic lesions is based on hypointense luminal filling defects with this approach. Water spiked with paramagnetic contrast is used to distend the bowel lumen and to render the lumen bright.[7,24–26] Most bright-lumen MR colonography strategies only administer high-signal contrast material rectally[25–29]; however, a few studies also added a paramagnetic oral contrast agent to the major meals before MR colonography to tag fecal residue, thereby ensuring homogeneous high signal throughout the bowel segments.[24,30,31] The downside of bright-lumen MR colonography is potential false-positive filling defects, caused by air or residual stool (**Boxes 2 and 3**).

In dark-lumen colonography a contrast agent with low signal intensity such as water, room air, or carbon dioxide is used to distend the colon, and an intravenous contrast agent allows visualization of the colonic wall and its pathology. Precontrast and postcontrast data acquisition is performed to differentiate between enhanced lesions and nonenhanced fecal material, thereby decreasing the false-positive and false-negative findings. Although preliminary studies focused on the bright-lumen approach, a change to dark-lumen imaging has occurred and is preferred, owing to the costs of the contrast agents for bowel distension in the bright-lumen approach and the false-positive findings of filling defects caused by air and residual stool.[27,32]

Box 1
Prerequisites of MR colonography

- Adequate colonic distension
- Bowel preparation with fecal tagging; either cathartic cleansing or more limited bowel preparation
- Spasmolytics to reduce bowel motion and bowel-motion artifacts
- Data acquisition during acceptable breath-hold times (15–20 seconds) to reduce breathing artifacts

Box 2
Pearls, pitfalls, and variants

Pearls:

- No use of ionizing radiation
- High soft-tissue contrast

Pitfalls:

- A collapsed colonic lumen impedes evaluation of the bowel lumen
- A collapsed colonic lumen can mimic colonic masses, resulting in false-positive findings
- Fecal residue can also mimic colonic masses, resulting in false-positive findings
- Flat lesions are a challenge for colonography and often result in false-negative findings

Variants:

- Bright-lumen MR colonography whereby the colon lumen has high signal intensity and the colonic wall low signal intensity
- Dark-lumen MR colonography whereby the colon lumen is low in signal intensity and the colonic wall has high signal intensity after administration of an intravenous paramagnetic contrast agent
- Bowel preparation with fecal tagging; either a limited preparation or cathartic cleansing
- Colonic distension can be established by water containing distending agents or gaseous distending agents (air or carbon dioxide)

Sequences and Field Strength

For both bright- and dark-lumen MR colonography, 3-dimensional (3D) T1-weighted gradient echo is commonly used (**Table 1**).[10] This sequence has a high spatial resolution with isotropic voxel size, providing multiplanar reconstruction (**Fig. 2**). Often a 2-dimensional (2D) T2-weighted half-Fourier acquisition single-shot turbo spin-echo

Box 3
Differential diagnosis of colorectal carcinoma on MR colonography

- Diverticulitis
- Inflammatory bowel disease
- Air or residual stool
- Lipoma
- Complex ileocecal valve
- Hemorrhoid

Table 1
Imaging protocols

	Coronal 3D T1-Weighted Turbo Field-Echo (TFE)	Coronal 2D T2-Weighted Half-Fourier Single-Shot Turbo Spin-Echo (HASTE)
Repetition time (ms)	2.2	800
Echo time (ms)	1.0	65
Flip angle (°)	10	90
Slice thickness (mm)	2	4
No. of signal averages	1	1
Fat saturation	Yes	No
Gap (mm)	—	1
Matrix	200 × 200	256 × 200
Field of view	400 × 400	400 × 400

Imaging parameters for dark-lumen 3.0-T MR colonography using a 3D T1-weighted TFE for lesion detection and 2D T2-weighted HASTE for problem solving.

(HASTE) or 2D T2-weighted true fast imaging with steady-state precession is also acquired (**Fig. 3**, see **Table 1**). These sequences are relatively insensitive for motion and susceptibility artifacts; lesion detection is modest, but the T2-weighted sequences can be used for problem solving (eg, insufficient image quality of T1-weighted images because of motion artifacts).

Both breathing and bowel motion can hamper the image quality. To avoid breathing artifacts, data should be acquired during breath-holds. Short repetition and echo times are required for data acquisition during acceptable breath-hold times (15–20 seconds) (see **Box 1**). Spasmolytics reduce bowel motion, which is essential for bowel imaging (see **Box 1**). Moreover, bowel distension may cause discomfort owing to bowel cramping, which is also reduced after administration of a spasmolytic agent. Glucagon and butylscopalamine are the most frequently used spasmolytics, usually administered intravenously for better control over the onset of the spasmolytics. However, half-life time is short, so careful timing of data acquisition is important. Butylscopalamine has been shown to result in better distension for CT colonography with carbon dioxide insufflation and lower patient burden. Moreover, overall patient burden on CT colonography was significantly lower for butylscopalamine,[33] although butylscopalamine is not approved by the US Food and Drug Administration for this indication.

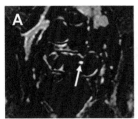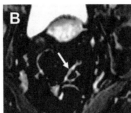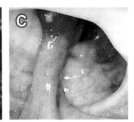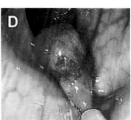

Fig. 2. Three-dimensional (3D) T1-weighted reconstruction. Dark-lumen MR colonography in a 61-year-old female patient. (*A*) Coronal 3D T1-weighted turbo field-echo showed a small enhanced lesion in the middle of the lumen of the sigmoid over several image slices. (*B*) Axial reconstruction clearly showed the stalk and head of a pedunculated polyp of 16 mm in the sigmoid. (*C, D*) Colonoscopy demonstrated a pedunculated polyp of 15 mm, which proved to be a tubular adenoma at histopathology.

For MR colonography, 1.5-T or higher MR fields are used for a homogeneous signal of the abdomen. A field strength of 1.5 T is the most frequently used in evaluation by MR colonography. Although the signal-to-noise ratio is higher in 3-T MR colonography, other implications of 3-T imaging, for example, specific absorption rate of energy, chemical shift artifacts, and prolonged relaxation times, hamper a 2-fold increase. A few studies have evaluated MR colonography with 3-T field strength in both phantom models[34,35] and human subjects (**Table 2**).[24,31,35–37] Saar and colleagues[37] demonstrated a per-patient sensitivity and specificity of 100% for lesions larger than 5 mm, and Graser and colleagues[36] showed a per-patient sensitivity and specificity of 90.9% and 98.5% for adenomas larger than 10 mm. However, it should be noted that similar results were also achieved with 1.5-T MR colonography.[38]

A large phased-array coil is used to cover the complete abdomen. However, in the authors' previous experience the field of view of the scanner (40 × 40 cm) did not always cover all colonic segments, therefore imaging of the upper abdomen and lower abdomen separately was preferred.

One image of the colon as a whole could be created with MR imaging system postprocessing software by fusion of the separate cranial and caudal stacks (**Fig. 4**). However, newer MR scanners have a larger field of view of (45 × 45 cm).

Parallel imaging can increase spatial resolution and decrease the scan time.

Dual Positioning

For dark- and bright-lumen imaging, dual positioning is recommended. For bright-lumen imaging in particular, dual positioning is necessary to differentiate between a colonic lesion and residual stool or air (**Fig. 5**). For dark-lumen imaging this is less essential because of precontrast and postcontrast imaging; however, dual positioning improves overall bowel distension. For both methods an optimal preparation of the bowel is essential, described in more detail below. Several studies on MR colonography performed data acquisition in one position only to reduce scan time. However, for CT colonography the acquisition of data in dual positions is standard.[18] The authors recommend dual positioning for MR colonography also.

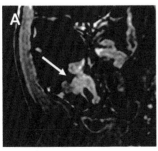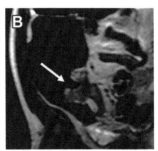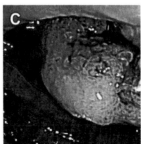

Fig. 3. Dark-lumen MR colonography of a 68-year-old male patient. Coronal 3D T1-weighted (*A*) turbo field-echo and 2-dimensional (2D) T2-weighted half-Fourier single-shot turbo spin-echo (*B*) demonstrated a (contrast-enhanced on T1-weighted sequence) mass lesion of 8 cm in the cecum, which was suspected to be colorectal cancer (*arrow*). (*C*) Colonoscopy detected a 4-cm mass lesion that was removed by hemicolectomy. Histopathology demonstrated a poorly differentiated adenocarcinoma, which originated from a tubulovillous adenoma.

Table 2
Overview of MR colonography studies on diagnostic accuracy of colorectal cancer detection in human subjects

Authors, Ref./Year	Bright or Dark Lumen MR Colonography	Bowel Preparation	Cleansing or Fecal Tagging	Colonic Distending Method	Field Strength (T)	Patient Population	No. of Patients
Luboldt et al,[7] 1997	Bright	Purged with water	Cleansing	Water/gadolinium mixture	1.5	NA	3
Luboldt et al,[26] 1998	Bright	PEG solution	Cleansing	Water/gadolinium mixture	1.5	First referral colonoscopy	23
Luboldt et al,[29] 2000	Bright	Preparation colonoscopy	Cleansing	Water/gadolinium mixture	1.5	Colonoscopy referral for excluding CRC	132
Pappalardo et al,[27] 2000	Bright	PEG solution	Cleansing	Water/gadolinium mixture	1.0	Large bowel obstruction	70
Saar et al,[28] 2000	Bright	Preparation colonoscopy	Cleansing	Water/gadolinium mixture	1.0	History polypectomy, FOBT+	5
Lauenstein et al,[39] 2001	Dark	Barium	Tagging	Barium/water mixture	1.5	Suspected CRC and volunteers	12[a]
Lauenstein et al,[32] 2001	Dark	PEG solution	Cleansing	Warm tap water	1.5	FOBT+ and family history	12
Morrin et al,[43] 2001	Both	Bisacodyl/sodium phosphate–based	Cleansing	Room air	1.5	NA	7
Lomas et al,[75] 2001	Dark	Sodium picosulfate, magnesium carbonate, citric acid–anhydrous	Cleansing	Carbon dioxide	1.5	Presence of CRC	7
Lauenstein et al,[14] 2002	Dark	Barium sulfate	Tagging	Warm tap water	1.5	Symptomatic patients	24

Ajaj et al,[44] 2003	Dark	PEG solution	Cleansing	Warm tap water	1.5	Variety of reasons for colonoscopy	122
Ajaj et al,[45] 2004	Dark	PEG solution	Cleansing	Room air or water	1.5	Variety of reasons for colonoscopy and 5 volunteers	55[b]
Lam et al,[46] 2004	Dark	Sodium phosphate solution	Cleansing	Room air	1.5	High-risk and average-risk patients	34
Leung et al,[59] 2004	Dark	Sodium phosphate solution or PEG solution	Cleansing	Room air	1.5	High-risk and average-risk patients	156[c]
Ajaj et al,[76] 2005	Dark	PEG solution	Cleansing	Warm tap water	1.5	Incomplete colonoscopy	37
Goehde et al,[40] 2005	Dark	Barium sulfate	Tagging	Warm tap water	1.5	Referral for colonoscopy	42
Lauenstein et al,[58] 2005	Dark and bright	PEG solution	Cleansing	Warm tap water	1.5	Suspected colorectal pathology	37
Hartmann et al,[77] 2005	Dark	PEG solution	Cleansing	Warm tap water	1.5	Incomplete colonoscopy	32
Hartmann et al,[48] 2006	Dark	PEG solution	Cleansing	Warm tap water	1.5	Symptomatic patients	92
Haykir et al,[78] 2006	Bright	NA	NA	NaCl/gadolinium mixture	1.5	FOBT+, rectal bleeding, altered bowel habits	33
Florie et al,[24] 2007	Bright	Lactulose, gadolinium	Tagging	Water/gadolinium mixture	1.5/3.0	Personal or family history of polyps and CRC	200
Kuehle et al,[42] 2007	Dark	Gastrografin, barium sulfate, locust bean gum	Tagging	Warm tap water	1.5	Screening population	315

(continued on next page)

Table 2
(continued)

Authors, Ref./Year	Bright or Dark Lumen MR Colonography	Bowel Preparation	Cleansing or Fecal Tagging	Colonic Distending Method	Field Strength (T)	Patient Population	No. of Patients
Saar et al,[25] 2007	Bright	PEG solution	Cleansing	Water/gadolinium mixture	1.5	Abdominal complaints, FOBT+, history of polypectomy	120
Saar et al,[37] 2008	Dark	PEG solution	Cleansing	Warm tap water	3.0	Scheduled for colonoscopy	34
Rodriguez Gomez et al,[38] 2008	Dark	Barium sulfate	Tagging	Water and room air	1.5	Clinical suspicion/ high risk	83
Achiam et al,[56] 2009	Dark	Barium sulfate/ ferumoxsil mixture	Tagging	Warm tap water	1.5	First-time referral colonoscopy	47
Achiam et al,[79] 2009	Dark	Sodium phosphate solution	Cleansing	Warm tap water	1.5	Proven rectal/ sigmoid cancer	46
Bakir et al,[61] 2009	Dark	Sodium phosphate solution	Cleansing	PEG-electrolyte solution[d]	1.5	Symptomatic patients	55
Keeling et al,[49] 2010	Dark	Sodium phosphate solution	Cleansing	Air	1.5	Screening and symptomatic	46
Sambrook et al,[60] 2012	NA	Barium sulfate	Tagging	Air	1.5	Scheduled for colonoscopy	29
Graser et al,[36] 2013	Dark	Bisacodyl, sodium phosphate, PEG solution	Cleansing	Warm tap water	3.0	Asymptomatic adults[e]	286

Abbreviations: CRC, colorectal carcinoma; FOBT+, positive fecal occult blood test; MRC, MR colonography; NA, not available; PEG, polyethylene glycol.
[a] 6 volunteers, 6 symptomatic patients.
[b] 50 patients, 5 volunteers.
[c] 76 average risk and 80 high risk.
[d] Oral administration only.
[e] 50 years or older with average risk and 40 years or older with a family history of colorectal cancer.

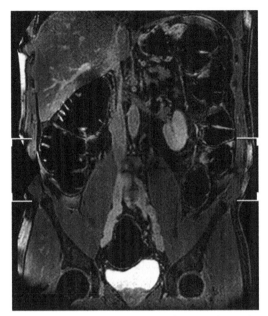

Fig. 4. Fusion of 2 separate stacks for complete colon evaluation. 3D T1-weighted turbo field-echo was acquired in 2 separate stacks of the upper and lower abdomen. After MR imaging, system postprocessing fusion of the stacks allowed evaluation of the complete colon.

Bowel Preparation

An overview on MR colonography studies and bowel preparations is summarized in **Table 2**.

Residual stool hampers an appropriate evaluation of the colon, as this can mimic intracolonic lesions (see **Boxes 2** and **3**). Therefore a bowel preparation is mandatory, consisting either of a full cathartic bowel cleansing or a less extensive bowel preparation with fecal tagging (see **Box 1** and **Table 2**). Bowel preparation with fecal tagging consists of modifying the signal intensity of feces, at either high signal intensity or low signal intensity; this helps to differentiate the colonic lumen from the colonic wall. Several tagging regimes have been proposed for both bright- and dark-lumen MR colonography, with the majority of studies evaluating barium-containing tagging agents.[14,39–42] First attempts at MR colonography prepared the patients with full cathartic bowel cleansing, as the MR colonography examination was immediately followed by colonoscopy.[26,27,43] For cathartic bowel cleansing, substances used for bowel purgation for colonoscopy, such as polyethyleneglycol-electrolyte solutions (PEG solutions) and sodium phosphate solutions, are generally applied. From colonoscopy it is known that full cathartic cleansing of the bowel leads to lower patient acceptance and participation in screening programs, and should therefore be avoided in MR colonography.[14] Nonetheless, most MR colonography diagnostic-accuracy studies use full cathartic bowel cleansing as a preparation regime, because the MR examinations are immediately followed by colonoscopy for comparison of the lesion detection.[25–27,32,36,44–49] Fecal tagging in combination with a limited bowel preparation instead of cathartic bowel cleansing, for example by adding a tagging contrast agent to principal meals 1 or 2 days before MR

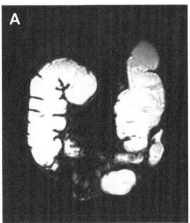
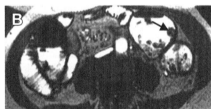
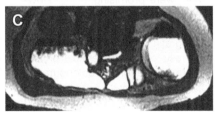

Fig. 5. Bright-lumen MR colonography of a 47-year-old female patient. After rectal administration of water spiked with a gadolinium-containing contrast agent, a coronal T1-weighted fast spoiled gradient echo demonstrated high signal intensity of the bowel lumen and low signal intensity of the colonic wall (*A*). Axial T1-weighted fast spoiled gradient echo without fat suppression showed presence of residual stool (*B*), which can mimic polyps (*arrow*). Dual positioning helps to overcome false-positive lesions as residual stool changes position by gravity (*C*).

colonography, increases patient acceptance.[50,51] From CT colonography it is known that a low-fiber diet the day before the MR colonography examination is essential for better tagged feces and better residue homogeneity, as dietary fibers are poorly digested by the gastrointestinal tract and thereby interfere with tagging regimes.[52,53]

An initial attempt at fecal tagging in MR colonography was performed in 2 healthy volunteers with oral administration of lactulose and simethicone, both with and without a gadolinium-based contrast agent for bright-lumen MR colonography, in combination with a gadolinium-containing enema.[30] As an alternative, to reduce costs related to the gadolinium-containing contrast agents, an oral barium-containing tagging agent (200 mg/mL 1 mg/mL barium sulfate with 4 principal meals) and barium-water mixture enema (1:4 barium/water) was evaluated for dark-lumen MR colonography in both healthy volunteers and patients.[38] Several studies showed that bowel preparation with barium-based fecal tagging was well tolerated and resulted in good image quality.[14,38,54]

These results, however, were in contradistinction to those of a different study using barium sulfate fecal tagging (150 mg/mL 1 mg/mL barium sulfate with 6 principal meals). Goehde and colleagues[40] demonstrated worse patient acceptance (mainly caused by painful constipation and stool thickening) compared with conventional colonoscopy. More importantly, Goehde and colleagues stopped including patients because of poor results of fecal tagging. Hence, lesion detection showed moderate results (1 lesion of 2 cm was detected, and for polyps, sensitivity was 40% for polyps of 10–19 mm and 16.7% for polyps of 6–9 mm). Moreover, a feasibility study on different preparation strategies demonstrated better patient acceptance for the strategy with gadolinium than with barium-based preparations.[55] Studies thereafter have aimed at improving their barium-based fecal tagging methods, as patients preferred MR colonography to colonoscopy and the detection rates were promising.[39,42,56] However, in a screening population with normal risk profile, fecal tagging with a solution (250 mL) containing 5% Gastrografin, 1% barium, and 0.2% locust bean gum resulted in an identical patient acceptance and preference for MR colonography and colonoscopy.[41,42] Moreover, a more recent study screening patients with average-risk and high-risk profiles preferred colonoscopy over MR colonography.[36] Patient acceptance and preference when undergoing colorectal examination is important for the study of screening patients, as patients' feeling of urgency to undergo a colorectal examination might differ from that of symptomatic patients, so that different patient acceptance and preferences might be expected.

The authors' group evaluated carbon dioxide rectal insufflation in combination with 4 bowel-preparation strategies consisting of gadolinium-based tagging, bowel purgation, barium-based tagging, and iodine-based tagging in 14 healthy volunteers. Residual stool volume was smallest in the bowel-purgation group and iodine-tagging group. In the latter, the bowel content was liquid owing to the laxative effect of the iodine tagging agent, and was rated as having slightly lower signal intensity when compared with the other preparation methods. The main advantage of iodine agents is the stool-softening effect, which ultimately leads to homogeneous tagging of the stool.[31,50] There was no significant difference in perceived burden between the 4 preparation strategies.[31]

In contrast to CT colonography whereby iodine- or barium-based tagging is standard practice, no consensus has been reached for bowel preparation in MR colonography.[18] Moreover, limited data are available on MR colonography bowel preparations in screening patients.[36,41,42] This aspect might be of interest, as one might expect differences in patient compliance between screening patients and high-risk patients. However, CT colonography data from a large, randomized controlled trial in a screening population showed good image quality, indicating that all screening patients had a high compliance to the iodine-tagging bowel preparation.[57]

Overall, the authors believe that a limited bowel preparation with fecal tagging (iodine or barium based) is important for future high patient acceptance of MR colonography as a screening tool for colorectal cancer. Therefore, future research on MR colonography for the detection of colorectal cancer should focus on minimizing the invasiveness of the bowel-preparation method. Furthermore, it should be emphasized that MR colonography with fecal tagging cannot be followed by immediate colonoscopy, as the colon is insufficiently cleansed.

Colon Distension

The second requisite for MR colonography is distension of the colon (see **Box 1**). The physiologic collapsed colon impedes evaluation of the intracolonic abnormality, as protruding masses and polyps may be concealed (see **Box 2**). Moreover, collapsed segments can mimic pathologic wall thickening; therefore colon luminal distension is required, with either water-based or air-based distending agents (see **Box 1**). In general, distension is provided by prone and supine positioning for optimal distension of all bowel segments. For example, optimal distension of the transverse colon is achieved in the supine position, whereas the rectum is best distended in prone position.

Initial efforts in MR colonography used rectal administration of a mixture of water with a paramagnetic contrast agent, which resulted in high signal intensity of the bowel lumen on T1-weighted sequences.[26–30] However, the mixture with a paramagnetic contrast agent was relatively expensive. Therefore, Lauenstein and colleagues[32] initiated bowel distension with a water-based enema only, resulting in a dark-lumen strategy.

In MR colonography with water-based distending agents, most studies use 2 to 2.5 L for bowel distension.[37,39,42,44,45,48,56,58] Water is administered by a rectal cannula under hydrostatic pressure. A drawback of this distending method is the potential spilling, embarrassment, and discomfort.[43]

A different method of colon distension is rectal administration of a gas. Either air or carbon dioxide can be used for bowel distension. This practice is common in CT colonography, whereby automated insufflation with carbon dioxide is the method of choice to maximize patient comfort and colonic distension.[18]

First attempts showed susceptibility artifacts, which hampered the image quality.[43] Improved imaging techniques enabled MR colonography distension by gaseous insufflation.[45] Ajaj and colleagues[45] demonstrated comparable distension for water-based and room air–based enemas. Susceptibility artifacts did not seem to be an issue. However, comparable discomfort was demonstrated for water-based and air-based distension in MR colonography.

Initial results from 36 patients using room-air distension for MR colonography were promising,[46] but the subsequent results from a larger study were disappointing, as it demonstrated interpretation difficulties owing to motion artifacts, and in this study patients preferred colonoscopy over MR colonography.[59] Moreover, polyp detection showed poor results (sensitivity 12.9% and specificity 97.6% for polyps >10 mm).

A different study also compared room-air distension with water-based distension in 83 patients.[39] Image quality showed significantly worse results for air-based distension regarding quality of distension and presence of artifacts. These differences were so evident that distension with room air was discontinued for the duration of the study. However, there was no significant difference in patient discomfort between air-based and water-based distension. In manual gaseous insufflation the intracolonic pressure might vary because of gas incontinence and ileocecal reflux, whereas in the case of water-based distension a constant distension of the colon is seen.

More recent studies have also evaluated the potential of colon distension with room air.[49,60] Sambrook and colleagues[60] demonstrated moderate results for diagnostic accuracy (sensitivity of 44% for lesions ≥10 mm) and image quality, whereas the groups of Keeling[49] demonstrated overall good image quality and high diagnostic accuracy. Patient preference for MR colonography, however, was equal to that of colonoscopy or even lower. This finding is in accordance with those of Leung and colleagues.[59] Both studies included high-risk and average-risk patients. The results for patient preference might be of interest for acceptance of MR colonography as a future screening tool.

Bakir and colleagues[61] evaluated MR colonography without additional rectal distension in 55 patients, who received an oral PEG solution for luminal distension over a 1- to 2-hour period. This study demonstrated adequate colonic distension in more than 91% of the patients. A drawback of the study was the prohibition for patients to defecate during preparation and examination, although no patients reported defecating involuntarily.

Regarding oral bowel preparation, there is no consensus for a bowel-distension method in MR colonography. The experience of carbon dioxide insufflation for MR colonography is fairly limited. From CT colonography it is known that carbon dioxide results in better distension of the sigmoid, transverse, and descending colon in the supine position, compared with insufflation of room air.[62] Furthermore, better patient acceptance was demonstrated for carbon dioxide insufflation compared with room-air insufflation.[63] The advantage of carbon dioxide insufflation is the reabsorption of the gas by the gastrointestinal tract, which causes less postprocedural discomfort arising from cramping and gas incontinence.[62,63] This reabsorption is not a limitation during the procedure when one uses continuous, automated insufflation with measurement of intracolonic pressure. Here loss of colonic filling will be supplemented by administration of carbon dioxide. Initial experience of carbon dioxide distension for MR colonography involved 7 patients with known colorectal carcinomas. The colon was insufflated by hand pressure and prefilled carbon dioxide containing enema bags. In all 7 patients the tumor was demonstrated, although additional administration of carbon dioxide was necessary in 1 patient because of inadequate luminal distension.

The authors' group also has evaluated the feasibility of carbon dioxide insufflation.[31] This study was the first to evaluate carbon dioxide distension by means of automated insufflation, as is standard practice in CT colonography. Automated insufflation for MR colonography has some practical issues, as there are no MR-compatible insufflators. Zijta and colleagues[31] tested an extended insufflation system with long tubing, to achieve maximum rectal pressure shutdown and prevent any pressure drop. Distension was adequate to optimal in 93% of the colon segments. Bowel-motion artifacts influenced image quality, but there was no association with susceptibility artifacts.

The authors believe that the future of MR colonography for the screening and diagnosis of colorectal cancer lies along the same pathway as for CT colonography, whereby automated carbon dioxide distending agents are used for colonic distension to reduce patient discomfort and provide for adequate colonic distension.

IMAGE EVALUATION

MR colonography data should be evaluated on a workstation that allows for reconstruction of the 3D-acquired datasets. As described earlier, for lesion detection the 3D T1-weighted sequences are used, and 2D T2-weighted sequences can be used for problem solving in cases of motion artifacts, inflammatory lesions, or extracolonic findings. Interpretation times are approximately 20 minutes.[49,61] Endoluminal fly-through can be helpful for polyp detection. Computer-aided detection (CAD) is known to increase the sensitivity of polyp detection on CT colonography without a decrease in specificity, but no data are available on the use of CAD in MR colonography examinations.[18] Both for CT colonography and MR colonography it is known that adequate training in image evaluation is necessary to achieve adequate detection rates.[64,65] For MR colonography no evidence is available regarding the minimum number of colonoscopy-verified cases to be evaluated for training to be considered adequate.

DIAGNOSTIC ACCURACY

As in CT colonography, MR colonography studies report colorectal lesion detection per lesion and per patient. Per-lesion analysis is a back-to-back comparison of the detected polyps at MR colonography with the colonoscopy results. Per-patient analysis provides information on detection rates of patients without any lesions and the detection rates of patients with 1 or more lesions present. This analysis is informative, as colonography is a triage technique in both screening and clinical practice. Here it is important that there is accurate triage, and the number of lesions is less important. Detection of colorectal carcinoma is the main focus of accurate detection in screening. For MR colonography, challenges lie in the distinction of mass lesions caused by colorectal cancer or by other pathologic conditions, such as diverticulitis or inflammatory bowel disease, which can mimic colorectal cancer masses (see **Box 3**; **Figs. 6** and **7**).

Furthermore, detection of large (>10 mm) and intermediate (6–9 mm) lesions are of interest in screening for colorectal cancer, and especially for its prevention. Diminutive lesions (<6 mm) are considered to be of lesser importance, as the chance of malignancy is very low.[66] From CT colonography data it is known that detection of flat lesions is challenging in comparison with pedunculated and sessile polyps.[67] For MR colonography, data on lesion detection rates for the different morphologic features are very limited and do not allow firm conclusions to be drawn.[25]

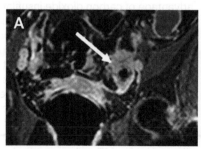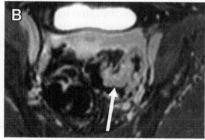

Fig. 6. Diverticulitis mimics colorectal cancer. Coronal (*A*) and axial (*B*) 3D T1-weighted turbo field-echo of a 64-year-old female patient demonstrated a poorly distended segment derived from stricture by a contrast-enhanced mass lesion in the sigmoid (*arrow*). The lesion was suspected to be colon carcinoma. Initial colonoscopy failed owing to lumen constriction. Hemicolectomy and histopathology showed extensive diverticulitis without any signs of malignancy.

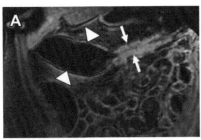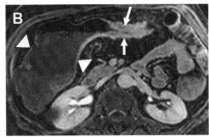

Fig. 7. Coronal (*A*) and axial (*B*) 3D T1-weighted turbo field-echo showed a stenotic segment (*arrows*) of 6 cm size with a prestenotic dilatation (*arrowheads*) in the transverse colon of a 53-year-old female patient, which was suspected to be Crohn disease, although colon carcinoma could not be ruled out. Histopathologic analysis after surgery showed a stenotic segment with inflammatory activity caused by Crohn disease.

A systematic review and meta-analysis was performed in 2010 at the authors' research department on MR colonography in the detection of colorectal lesions.[68] Thirteen studies were evaluated comprising a total of 1285 patients. The largest study (315 patients) included patients at average risk.[42] In 9 studies asymptomatic and/or symptomatic patients at increased risk of colorectal cancer were included,[14,24,25,37,40,48,58,59,69] whereas 3 studies did not describe indications for colonoscopy.[26,29,70] The meta-analysis demonstrated a sensitivity of 100% for the detection of colorectal carcinoma. Per-patient sensitivity and specificity estimates were 88% (95% confidence interval [CI] 63%–97%) and 99% (95% CI 95%–100%) for polyps with a size of 10 mm or larger. Per-polyp detection showed sensitivity of 84% (95% CI 66%–94%) for lesions larger than 10 mm. The diagnostic accuracy estimated for intermediate-sized lesions (6–9 mm) could not be calculated, because of the heterogeneity of the data. In this meta-analysis the highest per-polyp sensitivity of 6–9 mm was 86.2% (44 of 51)[25] and the lowest sensitivity was 16.7% (2 of 12),[40] and for polyps of 10 mm and larger the highest sensitivity was 100% in 2 studies (22 of 22) (9 of 9)[26,48] and the lowest per-polyp sensitivity 28.6% (2 of 7).[59]

The higher prevalence of abnormalities in high-risk patients will ultimately result in better diagnostic outcomes for sensitivity. The largest study in MR colonography was performed on 315 screening patients with normal risk profile.[42] Per-patient sensitivity was 60.0% for patients with polyps of 5 to 10 mm and increased to 70.0% for polyps larger than 10 mm. As described earlier, on a lesion basis a sensitivity of 62.2% for lesions larger than 5 mm and 73.9% for lesions larger than 10 mm was demonstrated.

A recent study published after the meta-analysis assessed MR colonography in 46 patients, both screening and symptomatic, after bowel cleansing and with room air distension.[49] This study demonstrated a per-patient sensitivity of 100% for polyps of 10 mm or larger and 6 mm or larger. When considering all sizes of polyps there was a per-patient sensitivity of 67% (95% CI 41.0%–86.6%) and specificity of 96.4% (95% CI 81.6%–99.9%).

Another recent study by Graser and colleagues[36] compared detection rates for advanced neoplasia of MR colonography in 286 asymptomatic adults. Advanced neoplasia is defined as colorectal neoplasia and advanced adenoma. Advanced adenoma was defined as an adenoma larger than 10 mm or showing either high-grade dysplasia or a prominent villous component. The rationale was that these lesions are the primary targets of colorectal screening. Patients underwent 3-T MR colonography after bowel purgation and room-air distension. The study demonstrated a sensitivity of 83.8% (95% CI 58.6%–96.4%) for patients with advanced neoplasia, and specificity of 95.3% (95% CI 91.9%–97.5%). The per-lesion detection of advanced neoplasia was 76.2% (95% CI 52.8%–91.8%).

Extracolonic Findings

MR colonography with high soft-tissue contrast enables extracolonic evaluation (**Fig. 8**). Ajaj and colleagues[71] reported 12% (31 subjects of 375) therapeutically relevant findings (according to the consensus proposal of extracolonic findings classification at CT colonography [Colonography Reporting and Data System][72]) in a dark-lumen study. Twenty-seven of 31 patients were subjected to additional examinations, and all findings were confirmed.[71] In a bright-lumen study a total of 10 findings (4.8%) were potentially therapeutically relevant, of which 2 were revealed to be malignant (1.0%). This study demonstrated high accuracy of MR colonography for extracolonic findings; however, the majority are of low clinical importance.[71,73] It remains to be shown whether

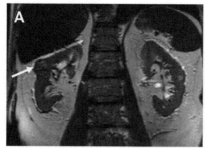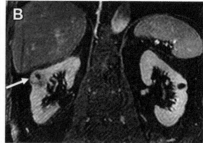

Fig. 8. Coronal 2D T2-weighted half-Fourier single-shot turbo spin-echo (*A*) and coronal 3D T1-weighted (*B*) turbo field-echo demonstrated a mass lesion of 2.6 by 2.7 cm (*arrow*) in the right kidney of a 58-year-old male patient. Histopathology demonstrated a renal cell carcinoma.

extracolonic findings are an asset or a liability with respect to cost-effectiveness and acceptance.

MR COLONOGRAPHY AND ITS FUTURE ROLE IN SCREENING

For MR colonography, extensive heterogeneity exists in study results regarding sensitivity and specificity values in the detection of colorectal lesions. This heterogeneity might be a consequence of variations in bowel preparations and distending agents, as well as in imaging techniques. More data on CT colonography are available regarding detection rates of colorectal cancer and polyps, in both average-risk and high-risk patients. CT colonography showed a per-patient sensitivity of 88% for advanced neoplasia of 10 mm or larger in screening populations and 96% for colorectal carcinoma in average-risk and high-risk populations.[11,12] For MR colonography a comparable per-patient sensitivity of 100% for colorectal carcinoma was found, and a sensitivity of 88% for lesions larger than 10 mm; however, these findings were in both high-risk and low-risk patients, most of whom were not screening patients.[68] Moreover, these estimates were calculated from a smaller

population than was evaluated with CT colonography. In addition, as detection rates differ among different readers, data on adequate training and CAD reading were evaluated for CT colonography, which is not available for MR colonography.[18] This weakness of MR colonography makes CT colonography a more viable alternative at present.

Cost-effectiveness will play a major role if MR colonography is to become a screening tool for colorectal cancer. For CT colonography, cost-effectiveness has been shown to be lower than for alternative methods, and CT colonography was estimated to be more cost-effective than colonoscopy if the unit costs were 60% of those of colonoscopy.[5] However, the results of these modeling studies were substantially influenced by the assumed costs of CT colonography. The first study on the actual costs of CT colonography in screening, which recently has been published, showed that the costs of an invitational-based CT colonography screening were €56.97 per invitee, €169.40 per participant, and €2772.51 per individual with detected advanced neoplasia.[74] This expense was substantially lower than the presumed costs used in the modeling studies. Further studies should look into the cost-effectiveness of CT colonography. There is no insight into the actual costs of an MR colonography–based screening program, and this information is mandatory before considering MR colonography as a screening tool for the detection of colorectal cancer (**Box 4**).

SUMMARY

MR colonography would be suited for screening for colorectal cancer because of its lack of ionizing radiation. However, no consensus has been reached regarding imaging sequences, bowel preparation, and colonic distension (see **Box 4**). Moreover, data on the diagnostic accuracy for polyp detection vary, and too little evidence on the diagnostic accuracy of MR colonography in screening populations is available (see **Box 4**).

Box 4
What the referring physician needs to know

- The results on diagnostic performance of MR colonography are promising but heterogeneous

- Thus far, MR colonography cannot be used as a colorectal screening tool

- The high soft-tissue contrast renders accurate extracolonic evaluation

- Data on cost-effectiveness of MR colonography are not available

- MR colonography should be evaluated in larger patient cohorts of screening patients

The available results are mediocre for medium-sized lesions, and inferior for this size category to results of CT colonography and, certainly, colonoscopy. Furthermore, data on cost-effectiveness, participation, compliance, and the pros and cons of extracolonic findings in screening are lacking (see **Box 4**). More insight into the optimal technique and associated accuracy measures are needed, as well as on the aforementioned issues such as cost-effectiveness, before MR colonography can be considered a viable option for screening.

MR colonography is not (yet) suited for screening for colorectal cancer (see **Box 4**). For now, MR colonography might be used in screening in rare cases where CT colonography or colonoscopy are contraindicated (eg, pregnancy) or in patients who refuse to undergo CT colonography and colonoscopy. Future research should clarify whether MR colonography–based screening is a viable option.

REFERENCES

1. Ferlay J, Parkin DM, Steliarova-Foucher E. Estimates of cancer incidence and mortality in Europe in 2008. Eur J Cancer 2010;46(4):765–81.

2. Levin B, Lieberman DA, McFarland B, et al. Screening and surveillance for the early detection of colorectal cancer and adenomatous polyps, 2008: a joint guideline from the American Cancer Society, the US Multi-Society Task Force on Colorectal Cancer, and the American College of Radiology. Gastroenterology 2008;134(5):1570–95.

3. Siegel R, Desantis C, Virgo K, et al. Cancer treatment and survivorship statistics, 2012. CA Cancer J Clin 2012;62:220–41.

4. Zauber A, Stewart ET, Waye JD. Colonoscopic polypectomy and long-term prevention of colorectal-cancer deaths. N Engl J Med 2012;366(8):687–96.

5. De Haan MC, Halligan S, Stoker J. Does CT colonography have a role for population-based colorectal cancer screening? Eur Radiol 2012;22(7):1495–503.

6. Vining D. Virtual endoscopy: is it reality? Radiology 1996;200:30–1.

7. Luboldt W, Bauerfeind P, Steiner P, et al. Preliminary assessment of three-dimensional magnetic resonance imaging for various colonic disorders. Lancet 1997;349(9061):1288–91.

8. Harewood GC, Wiersema MJ, Melton LJ. A prospective, controlled assessment of factors influencing acceptance of screening colonoscopy. Am J Gastroenterol 2002;97(12):3186–94.

9. Laghi A, Rengo M, Graser A, et al. Current status on performance of CT colonography and clinical indications. Eur J Radiol 2013;82(8):1192–200. http://dx.doi.org/10.1016/j.ejrad.2012.05.026.

10. Thornton E, Morrin MJ. Current status of MR colonography. Radiographics 2010;30:201–18.

11. De Haan MC, Van Gelder RE, Graser A, et al. Diagnostic value of CT-colonography as compared to colonoscopy in an asymptomatic screening population: a meta-analysis. Eur Radiol 2011;21(8):1747–63.

12. Pickhardt PJ, Hassan C, Halligan S, et al. Colorectal cancer: CT colonography and colonoscopy for detection—systematic review and meta-analysis. Radiology 2011;259(2):393–405.

13. Van Dam L, Kuipers EJ, Steyerberg EW, et al. The price of autonomy: should we offer individuals a choice of colorectal cancer screening strategies? Lancet Oncol 2013;14(1):38–46.

14. Lauenstein TC, Goehde SC, Ruehm SG, et al. MR colonography with barium-based fecal tagging: initial clinical experience. Radiology 2002;223(1):248–54.

15. Boellaard TN, Venema HW, Streekstra GJ, et al. Effective radiation dose in CT colonography: is there a downward trend? Acad Radiol 2012;19(9):1127–33.

16. Brenner D, Georgsson M. Mass screening with CT colonography: should the radiation exposure be of concern? Gastroenterology 2005;129(1):328–37.

17. Iafrate F, Hassan C, Pickhardt PJ, et al. Portrait of a polyp: the CTC dilemma. Abdom Imaging 2010;35(1):49–54.

18. Neri E, Halligan S, Hellström M, et al. The second ESGAR consensus statement on CT colonography. Eur Radiol 2013;23(3):720–9. http://dx.doi.org/10.1007/s00330-012-2632-x.

19. Fidler J, Johnson C. Flat polyps of the colon: accuracy of detection by CT colonography and histologic significance. Abdom Imaging 2009;34(2):157–71.

20. Gupta N, Bansal A, Rao D, et al. Prevalence of advanced histological features in diminutive and small colon polyps. Gastrointest Endosc 2012;75(5):1022–30.

21. Noffsinger AE. Serrated polyps and colorectal cancer: new pathway to malignancy. Annu Rev Pathol 2009;4:343–64.

22. Leedham S, East JE, Chetty R. Diagnosis of sessile serrated polyps/adenomas: what does this mean for the pathologist, gastroenterologist and patient? J Clin Pathol 2013;66(4):265–8.

23. Van der Paardt MP, Zijta FM, Stoker J. MRI of the colon. Imag Med 2010;2(2):195–209.

24. Florie J, Jensch S, Nievelstein R, et al. MR colonography with limited bowel preparation compared with optical colonoscopy in patients at increased risk for colorectal cancer. Radiology 2007;243(1):122–31.

25. Saar B, Meining A, Beer A, et al. Prospective study on bright lumen magnetic resonance colonography

in comparison with conventional colonoscopy. Br J Rheumatol 2007;80(952):235–41.

26. Luboldt W, Steiner P, Bauerfeind P, et al. Detection with of mass lesions colonography: preliminary report. Radiology 1998;207:59–65.

27. Pappalardo G, Polettini E, Frattaroli FM, et al. Magnetic resonance colonography versus conventional colonoscopy for the detection of colonic endoluminal lesions. Gastroenterology 2000;119(2):300–4.

28. Saar B, Heverhagen J, Obst T, et al. Magnetic resonance colonography and virtual magnetic resonance colonoscopy with the 1.0 system. Invest Radiol 2000;35(9):521–6.

29. Luboldt W, Bauerfeind P, Wildermuth S, et al. Gastrointestinal imaging colonic masses: detection with MR Colonography. Radiology 2000;216:383–8.

30. Weishaupt D, Patak MA, Froehlich JM, et al. Faecal tagging to avoid colonic cleansing before MRI colonography. Lancet 1999;354(9181):835–6.

31. Zijta FM, Nederveen AJ, Jensch S, et al. Feasibility of using automated insufflated carbon dioxide (CO(2)) for luminal distension in 3.0T MR colonography. Eur J Radiol 2012;81(6):1128–33.

32. Lauenstein TC, Herborn CU, Vogt FM, et al. Dark lumen MR-colonography: initial experience. Rofo 2001;173(9):785–9.

33. De Haan MC, Boellaard TN, Bossuyt PM, et al. Colon distension, perceived burden and side effects of CT-colonography for screening using hyoscine butylbromide or glucagon hydrochloride as bowel relaxant. Eur J Radiol 2012;81(8):910–6.

34. Wessling J, Fischbach R, Borchert A, et al. Detection of colorectal polyps: comparison of multi–detector row CT and MR colonography in a colon phantom. Radiology 2006;241(1):125–31.

35. Rottgen R, Herzog H, Bogen P, et al. MR colonoscopy at 3.0 T: comparison with 1.5 T in vivo and a colon model. Clin Imaging 2006;30:248–53.

36. Graser A, Melzer A, Lindner E, et al. Magnetic resonance colonography for the detection of colorectal neoplasia in asymptomatic adults. Gastroenterology 2013;144(4):743–50.

37. Saar B, Gschossmann JM, Bonel HM, et al. Evaluation of magnetic resonance colonography at 3.0 Tesla regarding diagnostic accuracy and image quality. Invest Radiol 2008;43(8):580–6.

38. Rodriguez Gomez S, Pagés Llinas M, Castells Garangou A, et al. Dark-lumen MR colonography with fecal tagging: a comparison of water enema and air methods of colonic distension for detecting colonic neoplasms. Eur Radiol 2008;18(7):1396–405.

39. Lauenstein T, Holtmann G, Schoenfelder D, et al. MR colonography without colonic cleansing: a new strategy to improve patient acceptance. AJR Am J Roentgenol 2001;177:823–7.

40. Goehde SC, Descher E, Boekstegers A, et al. Dark lumen MR colonography based on fecal tagging for detection of colorectal masses: accuracy and patient acceptance. Abdom Imaging 2005;30(5):576–83.

41. Kinner S, Kuehle CA, Langhorst J, et al. MR colonography vs optical colonoscopy: comparison of patients' acceptance in a screening population. Eur Radiol 2007;17(9):2286–93.

42. Kuehle CA, Langhorst J, Ladd SC, et al. Magnetic resonance colonography without bowel cleansing: a prospective cross sectional study in a screening population. Gut 2007;56(8):1079–85.

43. Morrin MM, Hochman MG, Farrell RJ, et al. MR colonography using colonic distention with air as the contrast material: work in progress. AJR Am J Roentgenol 2001;176(1):144–6.

44. Ajaj W. Dark lumen magnetic resonance colonography: comparison with conventional colonoscopy for the detection of colorectal pathology. Gut 2003;52(12):1738–43.

45. Ajaj W, Lauenstein TC, Pelster G, et al. MR colonography: how does air compare to water for colonic distention? J Magn Reson Imaging 2004; 19(2):216–21.

46. Lam WW, Leung WK, Wu JKL, et al. Screening of colonic tumors by air-inflated magnetic resonance (MR) colonography. J Magn Reson Imaging 2004; 19(4):447–52.

47. Lim EJ, Leung C, Pitman A, et al. Magnetic resonance colonography for colorectal cancer screening in patients with Lynch syndrome gene mutation. Fam Cancer 2010;9(4):555–61.

48. Hartmann D, Bassler B, Schilling D, et al. Colorectal polyps: detection with dark lumen MRC versus conventional colonoscopy. Radiology 2006;238(1):143–9.

49. Keeling AN, Morrin MM, McKenzie C, et al. Intravenous, contrast-enhanced MR colonography using air as endoluminal contrast agent: impact on colorectal polyp detection. Eur J Radiol 2010;81:31–8.

50. Liedenbaum MH, Denters MJ, Zijta FM, et al. Reducing the oral contrast dose in CT colonography: evaluation of faecal tagging quality and patient acceptance. Clin Radiol 2011;66(1):30–7.

51. Florie J, Birnie E, Van Gelder RE, et al. MR colonography with limited bowel preparation: patient acceptance compared with that of full-preparation colonoscopy. Radiology 2007;245(1):150–9.

52. Liedenbaum MH, Denters MJ, De Vries AH, et al. Low-fiber diet in limited bowel preparation for CT colonography: influence on image quality and patient acceptance. AJR Am J Roentgenol 2010; 195(1):31–7.

53. Chen H, Haack VS, Janecky CW, et al. Mechanisms by which wheat bran and oat bran increase stool. Am J Clin Nutr 1998;68(3):711–9.

54. Papanikolaou N, Grammatikakis J, Maris T, et al. MR colonography with fecal tagging: comparison

between 2D turbo FLASH and 3D FLASH sequences. Eur Radiol 2003;13(3):448–52.

55. Florie J, Van Gelder RE, Haberkorn B, et al. Magnetic resonance colonography with limited bowel preparation: a comparison of 3 strategies. J Magn Reson Imaging 2007;25(4):766–74.

56. Achiam MP, Løgager VB, Chabanova E, et al. Diagnostic accuracy of MR colonography with fecal tagging. Abdom Imaging 2009;34(4):483–90.

57. Stoop EM, De Haan MC, De Wijkerslooth TR, et al. Participation and yield of colonoscopy versus non-cathartic CT colonography in population-based screening for colorectal cancer: a randomised controlled trial. Lancet Oncol 2012;13(1):55–64.

58. Lauenstein TC, Ajaj W, Kuehle CA, et al. Magnetic resonance colonography: comparison of contrast-enhanced 3-dimensional vibe with 2-dimensional FISP sequences. Invest Radiol 2005;40(2):89–96.

59. Leung WK, Lam WW, Wu JC, et al. Magnetic resonance colonography in the detection of colonic neoplasm in high-risk and average-risk individuals. Am J Gastroenterol 2004;99(1):102–8.

60. Sambrook A, Mcateer D, Yule S, et al. MR colonography without bowel cleansing or water enema: a pilot study. Br J Radiol 2012;85(1015):921–4.

61. Bakir B, Acunas B, Bugra D, et al. MR colonography after oral administration of polyethylene glycol-electrolyte solution. Radiology 2009;251(3):901–9.

62. Shinners TJ, Pickhardt PJ, Taylor AJ, et al. Patient-controlled room air insufflation versus automated carbon dioxide delivery for CT colonography. AJR Am J Roentgenol 2006;186(6):1491–6.

63. Sumanac K, Zealley I, Fox BM, et al. Minimizing postcolonoscopy abdominal pain by using CO insufflation: a prospective, randomized, double blind, controlled trial evaluating a new commercially available CO delivery system. Gastrointest Endosc 2002;56(2):190–4.

64. Zijta FM, Florie J, Jensch S, et al. Diagnostic performance of radiographers as compared to radiologists in magnetic resonance colonography. Eur J Radiol 2010;75(2):12–7.

65. Liedenbaum MH, Bipat S, Bossuyt PM, et al. Evaluation of a standardized CT colonography training program for novice readers. Radiology 2011; 258(2):477–87.

66. Lieberman DA, Rex DK, Winawer SJ, et al. Guidelines for colonoscopy surveillance after screening and polypectomy: a consensus update by the US Multi-Society Task Force on Colorectal Cancer. Gastroenterology 2012;143(3):844–57.

67. Pickhardt PJ, Wise SM, Kim DH. Positive predictive value for polyps detected at screening CT colonography. Eur Radiol 2010;20(7):1651–6.

68. Zijta FM, Bipat S, Stoker J. Magnetic resonance (MR) colonography in the detection of colorectal lesions: a systematic review of prospective studies. Eur Radiol 2010;20(5):1031–46.

69. Kerker J, Albes G, Roer N, et al. MR-colonography in hospitalized patients: feasibility and sensitivity. Z Gastroenterol 2008;46(4):339–43.

70. Achiam MP, Chabanova E, Løgager VB, et al. MR colonography with fecal tagging: barium vs barium ferumoxsil. Acad Radiol 2008;15(5):576–83.

71. Ajaj W, Ruehm SG, Ladd SC, et al. Utility of dark-lumen MR colonography for the assessment of extra-colonic organs. Eur Radiol 2007;17(6): 1574–83.

72. Zalis ME, Barish MA, Choi JR, et al. Radiology for the working group on virtual colonoscopy CT colonography reporting and data system: a consensus proposal. Radiology 2005;236(1):3–9.

73. Yusuf E, Florie J, Nio CY, et al. Incidental extracolonic findings on bright lumen MR colonography in a population at increased risk for colorectal carcinoma. Eur J Radiol 2011;78(1):135–41.

74. De Haan MC, Thomeer M, Stoker J, et al. Unit costs in population-based colorectal cancer screening using CT colonography performed in university hospitals in The Netherlands. Eur Radiol 2013; 23(4):897–907.

75. Lomas DJ, Sood RR, Graves MJ, et al. Colon carcinoma: MR imaging with CO_2 enema—pilot study. Radiology 2001;219(2):558–62.

76. Ajaj W, Lauenstein TC, Pelster G, et al. MR colonography in patients with incomplete conventional colonoscopy. Radiology 2005;234(9):452–9.

77. Hartmann D, Bassler B, Schilling D, et al. Incomplete conventional colonoscopy: magnetic resonance colonography in the evaluation of the proximal colon. Endoscopy 2005;37(9):816–20.

78. Haykir R, Karakose S, Karabacakoglu A, et al. Detection of colonic masses with MR colonography. Turk J Gastroenterol 2006;17(3):191–7.

79. Achiam MP, Holst Anderson LP, Klein M, et al. Preoperative evaluation of synchronous colorectal cancer using MR colonography. Acad Radiol 2009;16(7):790–7.

Magnetic Resonance Imaging of Rectal and Anal Cancer

Michael R. Torkzad, MD, PhD[a],*, Ihab Kamel, MD, PhD[b],
Vivek Gowdra Halappa, MD[b],
Regina G.H. Beets-Tan, MD, PhD[c]

KEYWORDS

- Rectum • Anus • Cancer • Magnetic resonance imaging • Staging

KEY POINTS

- Magnetic resonance imaging plays a pivotal role in the imaging and staging of rectal and anal carcinomas.
- For rectal adenocarcinomas assessment of tumor relation to mesorectal fascia, vessel involvement, relation to pelvic floor and neighboring organs are best assessed by MRI and important to report.
- A primary squamous cell or epidermoid carcinoma of the anatomic rectum has different staging and staged differently than rectal adenocarcinoma. Avery attempt should be made to characterize tumor size, growth into neighboring organs and lymph node staging correctly.

INTRODUCTION

Rectal and anal cancers are malignancies of the gastrointestinal tract with important health implications. Rectal cancer deserves special attention because of its high associated mortality, although recently, at least in some countries, the mortality rate after rectal cancer has been reduced, mostly because of improved local management of disease, which is attributed at least in part to multidisciplinary team (MDT) meetings and pelvic magnetic resonance (MR) imaging. The local recurrence rate for rectal cancer, which was 30% to 40% a few decades ago, is now less than 10%, and this has had an impact on survival in certain Western countries.[1–3] Anal cancer is much less common, with better survival rates (80% cure rate or 5-year survival). The staging and behavior of the 2 cancers is almost completely different. The most specific distinguishing features are histopathologic, not the location of the tumor as the names would suggest. A primary squamous cell or epidermoid carcinoma (SCC)[4] of the anatomic rectum should be treated and regarded as an anal cancer; whereas a primary adenocarcinoma of the anal canal is regarded as a rectal cancer (**Fig. 1**).

MR IMAGING OF PRIMARY RECTAL CANCER

Although radiology has been used for confirming colon cancer in cases with typical "apple-core" lesions, this approach is now used only for tumors inaccessible by endoscopic methods. Today, providing tissue samples for research and clinical analyses are necessary, and the role of MR imaging or any radiologic imaging method in the diagnosis of primary cancer is secondary in this

No relationships to disclose.
[a] Section of Radiology, Department of Radiology, Oncology and Radiation Science, Uppsala University, Uppsala 75185, Sweden; [b] Department of Radiology and Radiological Sciences, The Johns Hopkins University School of Medicine, 600 N. Wolfe Street, Baltimore, MD 21287, USA; [c] Department of Radiology, Maastricht University Medical Center, PO Box 5800, Maastricht 6202 AZ, The Netherlands
* Corresponding author.
E-mail address: michael.torkzad@gmail.com

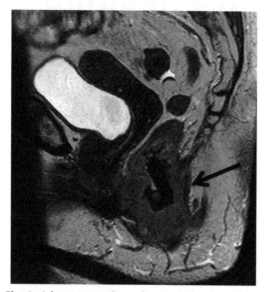

Fig. 1. A large tumor (*arrow*) extending anteriorly to female vestibule and introitus. The decision to regard this as low rectal cancer or anal cancer depends on histopathology, which showed that the tumor is squamous cell carcinoma. The treatment and staging is therefore based on anal cancer.

regard. This fact is especially true in rectal cancer, where the tumor is easier to reach than the more oral parts of the colon. However, there are occasions when MR imaging and/or other imaging modalities must provide support for the diagnosis.[5] These situations arise mostly on the following occasions:

1. When repeated biopsies fail to provide a sign of malignancy in a highly suspicious lesion (**Fig. 2**)
2. When a stricture obstructs the endoscopic approach

In the case of a visible lesion, every effort is made to repeat the biopsies and to provide sufficient tissue samples. However, MR imaging can occasionally be of help. In tumors with clear signs of malignancy such as unequivocal extramural growth, mucin production, or malignant perirectal lymph nodes, a presumptive work hypothesis of rectal cancer can be made. However, the authors do not recommend this approach unless the members of the MDT understand the limitations of such a diagnosis and the radiologist is highly experienced.

There are also times when a lesion is not clearly visible. As already mentioned, the typical rectal cancer is an adenocarcinoma. These tumors arise from the mucosal layer, and if untreated they should be always visible from the luminal side.

However, some tumors such as gastrointestinal stromal tumors (GISTs) commonly arise from the outer bowel wall layers (**Fig. 3**). GISTs may ulcerate the mucosal layer, but sometimes biopsies of these lesions prove difficult. A radiologist can provide some clue to this diagnosis.

Strictures sometimes make negotiating the colon impossible. This scenario usually occurs in patients with strictures caused by diverticulitis, fibrotic adhesions, or peritoneal implants. These strictures are usually located at the rectosigmoid junction or higher up in the sigmoid colon (**Fig. 4**). The possible advantages of MR imaging are the feasibility of distinguishing low signal intensity (SI) thickened muscle wall layer from tumors that have intermediate to high SI, and the easier distinction of abscess from large mucin tumors. Review of previous images can be extremely helpful (**Fig. 5**).

The role of MR imaging of rectal cancer can be categorized in the following ways:

1. To stage a primary rectal cancer, the most widely accepted role
2. To evaluate preoperative response
3. To help diagnosis and/or evaluate local recurrence

Staging a Primary Rectal Cancer

The "holy plane"

The mesorectal fascia (MRF) is the most important surgical landmark alongside growth into neighboring organs for the planning of a surgical approach. Involvement of the MRF is associated with a high rate of local recurrence. Heald and Ryall[6] introduced the concept of removing the whole mesorectal compartment including the rectal cancer, which resulted in a significant reduction of local recurrence rates in rectal cancer. MRF is a thin layer of connective tissue surrounding the perirectal fat, seen as a dark thin layer separating the perirectal fat from neighboring structures (**Fig. 6**). It is also seen on computed tomography (CT), but not on endoanal or transabdominal ultrasonography. The fact that MRF is seen on CT can make CT a useful compromise when MR imaging cannot be performed, such as in cases of claustrophobia or pacemaker (**Fig. 7**). However, for lower rectal tumors, CT is much less helpful.

One has to note that MRF and the circumferential resection margin (CRM) are not the same. MRF is defined anatomically; whereas CRM is determined by the how the surgical procedure has been performed. CRM can be inside as well outside MRF. The role of pelvic MR imaging is to alert the surgeon and MDT of threatened MRF.[7]

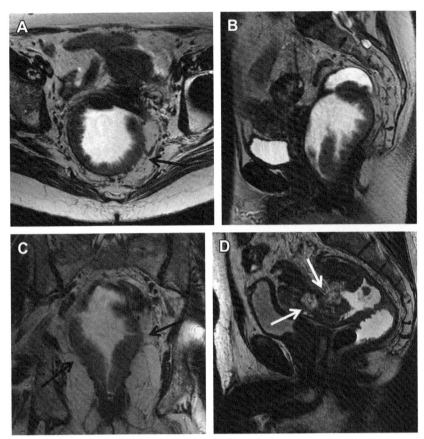

Fig. 2. (*A–C*) Benign villous adenoma in a female patient. Several biopsies fail to show signs of malignancy. However, MR imaging was performed because the request was written before histopathologic results were known shows areas with suspected breach or at least hazy muscular propria (*black arrows*). The first radiologist therefore assigned a T3 stage. At a multidisciplinary team (MDT) meeting, however, this was retracted and changed to "no definitive signs of malignancy" by the senior radiologist, which was confirmed later after surgery. It is noteworthy that T staging is only for malignant tumors, and therefore stage T1 should never be used for benign tumors. (*D*) Sagittal image from another patient also showing a polypoid tumor with intussusception. Intussusception makes assessment of extramural growth difficult. However, a mucin component (*white arrows*) is a sign of malignancy.

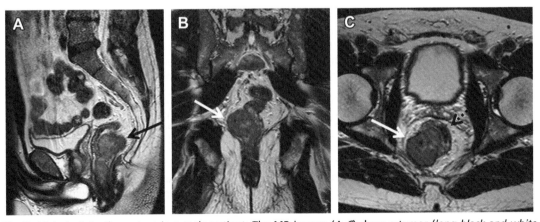

Fig. 3. Metastasis to the rectum in a male patient. The MR images (*A–C*) show a tumor (*long black and white arrows*) that was causing symptoms. However, this tumor was not seen by the endoscopist probably because of an intact lumen. The axial image shows best how the mucosal layer of rectum (*short dotted arrow in C*) is lifted up by the tumor. Note that in the case of metastases the discussion is seldom about mesorectal fascia or T staging.

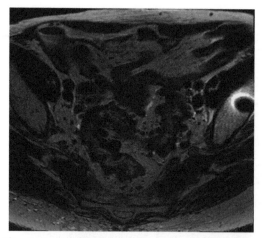

Fig. 4. Typical features of diverticular disease in a patient who could not have complete sigmoidoscopy. CT of the colon (not shown) shows thickened wall of the sigmoid not fully expanded on neither prone nor supine images. MR imaging helps one to appreciate the hypertrophied muscular wall of the colon, which is of lower signal intensity (SI) than that of a tumor. No tumor is seen on MR imaging.

Threatened MRF is defined by how close the tumor is to MRF. Various margins have been selected from 1 to 5 mm; 1 mm or less constitutes threatened margin.[8] When a tumor traverses through MRF or leads to an unequivocal thickening of MRF, MRF is involved. For most radiologists threatened MRF and involved MRF are considered synonymous, and patients will undergo similar treatment stratification.

It is noteworthy that sometimes a satellite metastasis (discontinuous tumor) or lymph node metastasis can be close to the MRF. In the case of lymph node metastasis, it is the metastatic part of the node that can threaten MRF. Based on recent suggestions by Brown's group,[9] one needs to be less inclined to call MRF threatened if a lymph node is close to or abutting MRF, unless the node shows signs of malignancies and capsule breach (Figs. 8 and 9).

MRF is tethered closely to the parietal pelvic fasciae on pelvic side walls.[10] These fasciae merge into presacral fascia, which is in front of sacrum and the retroperitoneal vessels adjacent to sacrum. Lower down, the MRF covers the pelvic musculature (ie, levator ani muscles). Higher up, as rectum becomes completely peritoneal and sigmoid colon starts, MRF loosens from parietal pelvic and presacral fasciae and follows the superior rectal artery. At the highest point of its attachment to pelvic side walls, the MRF has been regarded as the uterosacral ligament in females. Just above

this is the peritoneal cavity, therefore peritoneal implants and endometriosis often tend to be seen here. Ventrally MRF lies behind the vagina and cervix in females and the prostate and seminal vesicles in males. Lower down, MRF is fused to Denovilliers fascia in male subjects. Higher up, as rectum becomes covered anteriorly by peritoneum, MRF disappears. Here no CRM is defined and, therefore, MRF is considered absent. When the serosal surface and, consequently, the peritoneal cavity are present, no CRM is defined; this is applicable to both rectum and colon. Therefore, one should defer from measuring the distance to serosal surface as a substitute for distance to MRF.

Low rectal tumors

For low rectal tumors the system devised by Shihab and colleagues[9] should be used (Fig. 10). Here the most important surgical plane is the intersphincteric plane, a fatty plane seen between the internal and external sphincters below, and the puborectalis muscle/levator muscle and muscularis propria higher up.[11] This approach is very practical, as measuring the distances is extremely difficult. A tumor-free intersphincteric plane ensures safe surgical resection. One should recall that the internal sphincter is basically a continuation of (circular layer of) the muscularis propria.

Adjacent organs

Growth into neighboring organ constitutes T4 based on the TNM classification (Figs. 11 and 12).[12] Most studies, though reporting high accuracy rates for T4 designation, do not distinguish between different organs. The soft-tissue contrast provided by MR imaging enables the clinician to provide precise T4-staging. One has to remember that simple proximity of tumor to an adjacent organ does not necessarily translate into tumor growth (T4 status). The authors recommend review of all available sequences to rule out (or rule in) growth into neighboring organs. This approach should not be limited to MR imaging only. Occasionally the authors have had help from reviewing CT colonography images, as these are obtained in 2 bodily positions perhaps with a different amount of urine in the bladder. If a near simultaneous image shows tumor and neighboring organ moving away from each other with the appearance of a clear fatty interspace, there is less likelihood of T4 stage. Conversely, close proximity on all images and positions could be a sign of a threatened organ invasion.

Previous TNM classifications designated perforation at the site of the tumor as T4. This clarification is omitted in TNM7, and the question is raised

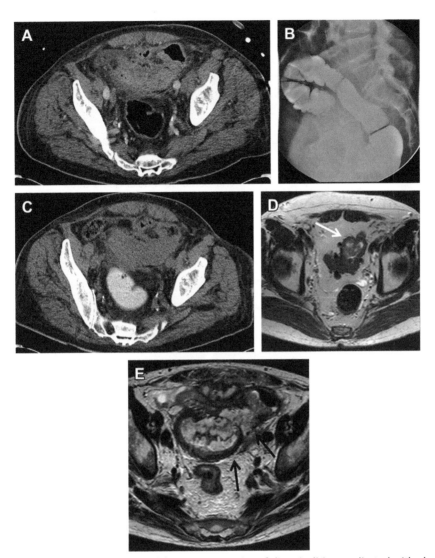

Fig. 5. A male patient presents with clinical features suggestive of diverticulitis complicated with abscess formation in November 2011. Twelve CT scans (*A*) over a period of 3 weeks show progressive disease. A sigmoidoscopy fails to negotiate to the area of interest. A contrast enema (*B*) followed by CT (*C*) is inconclusive. Ultrasound fine-needle aspiration yields no conclusive results. Finally the case is brought to an MDT meeting, despite no cancer diagnosis. A review of any possibly relevant past imaging is done. On 2 upper axial sections of an MR image of the prostate performed in April 2010 (*D*), a previous missed polyp (*white arrow*) is noted in the same area. A current MR image (*E*) shows the mucinous tumor clearly (*black arrows*).

about classification of tumor perforations. Perforations of the serosal layer are still considered T4a and not T4b. Fortunately tumor perforations are rare, especially in the rectum (**Fig. 13**).

Three areas demand extra attention:

1. Organs anterior to the rectum
2. Pelvic floor
3. Serosal layer

Organs anterior to rectum The amount of fat anterior to rectum is the least amount of fat surrounding the sides of the rectum, especially in female subjects (**Fig. 14**). Although no correlation between the total mesorectal volume and radiologic staging inaccuracy has been shown, the highest tumor overstaging has traditionally involved organs ventral to the rectum. Imaging in planes perpendicular to the interface of anterior rectal

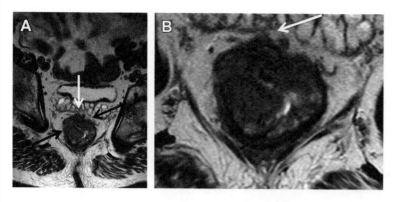

Fig. 6. (*A*) Image perpendicular to the rectum at the level of tumor (*black arrows*). The tumor is closest (*white arrows*) ventrally to the anterior part of mesorectal fascia, with almost clear fat intervention shown on the enlarged view of the same image (*B*).

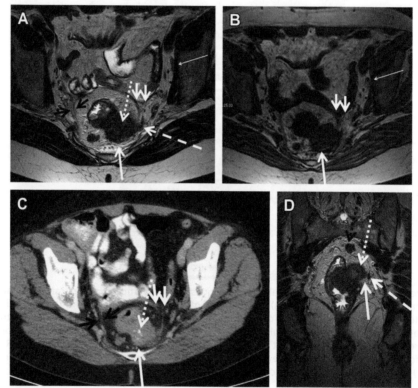

Fig. 7. A T3 tumor in a male patient. Axial T2-weighted (*A*), axial T1-weighted (*B*), axial contrast-enhanced CT (*C*), and coronal T2-weighted (*D*) images are shown, demonstrating that adequate assessment involves using all available imaging. While T2-weighted imaging provides the best soft-tissue contrast, the abundant perirectal/mesorectal fat helps one to see the tumor outgrowth clearly on T1- and T2-weighted images and on CT images (*thick long white arrows*). This tumor involves the mesorectal fascia, and might be responsible for separation of mesorectal (proper perirectal) fascia from visceral parietal fascia (*short thick white arrows*). Note that these fasciae are also separated ventrally on the right side (*short black arrows*). The calcification seen on CT image (*dotted white arrow*) is seen as black areas inside the tumor on T2-weighted images (*dotted white arrows*) and lymph node (*black dotted arrow in D*). Calcifications are seldom seen in combination with mucin (best appreciated on image *D*) and are a very specific sign of metastasis from adenocarcinomas. The short dashed arrow is a perineural tumor growth often missed on imaging. However, growth alongside visceral pelvic fascia should raise suspicion of such tumors. Such large tumors might metastasize to pelvic side walls. The node behind external iliac vessels (*thin white arrow*), however, is symmetric to the contralateral part, and its fatty hilum is better shown on a T1-weighted image.

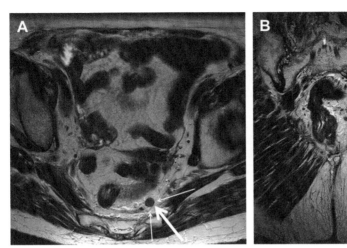

Fig. 8. Axial (*A*) and coronal (*B*) T2-weighted images of a patient with rectal cancer. One particular lymph node (*white thick arrows*) is particularly close to the mesorectal fascia (*thin arrows*) on the axial image. This node has a smooth border (in favor of benignity), is relatively large (somewhat in favor of malignancy), and shows heterogeneity especially on the coronal image (favors malignancy). This node was read as malignant, which was confirmed at histopathology. However, this node does not threaten mesorectal fascia.

wall and these organs might overcome overestimation of tumor growth ventrally. 3D imaging has shown some promise in terms of demonstrating clean fat space that might otherwise be missed.[13]

Pelvic floor The somewhat round rectum ampulla is situated just above the funnel-shaped pelvic floor. Because the pelvic floor forms an angled plane in relation to orthogonal coronal and axial

planes, with such nonanatomic imaging planes partial volume effect becomes very striking in this area, probably explaining why the pelvic floor is the second most commonly overstaged nearby organ. The best imaging plane to resolve such a problem would be perpendicular to the pelvic floor. Empty rectum could help reduce the roundness of the ampulla and increase the distance between the pelvic floor and rectal wall, thus

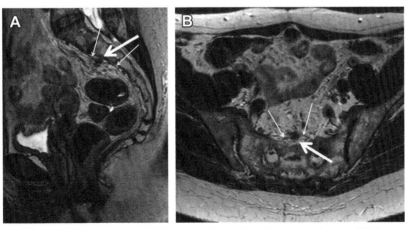

Fig. 9. A patient with stage T1 tumor (not visible) and malignant lymph node metastasis (*thick arrows*) on sagittal (*A*) and axial (*B*) T2-weighted images. This malignant lymph node is very irregular in contour, and is somewhat enlarged and heterogeneous. It also involves the dorsal part of mesorectal fascia, which is fused to the presacral fascia (*thin arrows*).

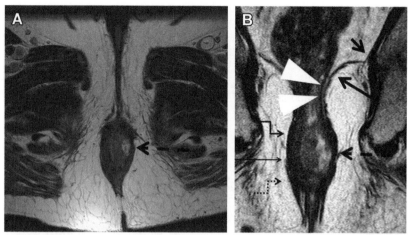

Fig. 10. A low rectal tumor seen on axial (*A*) and coronal (*B*) T2-weighted images. This tumor has mucin component (*dashed arrows*) and therefore shows high SI. The fact that it pushes the anal canal makes its assessment difficult. The levator ani muscles (*long solid black arrow*) originate from the fascia covering the internal obturator muscles (*short black arrow*). It becomes more thickened, especially in men, and this part forms the puborectal muscle (*crooked solid arrow*). The puborectal muscle contributes to the sphincter function even though it is not anatomically the same muscle. Usually there is some gap (*long thin solid arrow*) between this muscle and the external sphincter muscle (*crooked dotted arrow*), probably explaining why anal fistulas choose this gap for further extension. The continuation of muscularis propria (*large white arrowheads*) becomes the internal sphincter. In this patient no discernible fat is seen between the internal and external sphincter complexes and therefore a larger excision is planned.

reducing partial volume effect. As observed on any CT colonogram, the ampulla tends to efface the rectum against the pelvic floor and surrounding MRF. Rectum expansion is thus not recommended.

Tumors in the ampulla, both benign and malignant, might become large in the luminal portion (**Fig. 15**). This rectum expansion, which behaves in the same way as rectal expansion caused by rectal balloon and enema, could lead to diagnostic

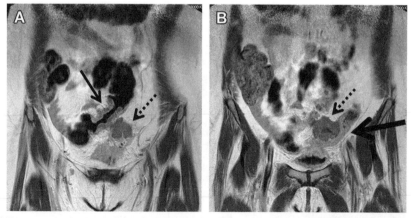

Fig. 11. (*A, B*) Two consecutive T1-weighted images without fat saturation, both after gadolinium enhancement. Note that the tumor initiates from one sigmoid loop (*solid arrow in A*), and shows an outgrowth (*dotted arrows*) that reaches another sigmoid loop (*large arrow*). Even though both involved loops are sigmoid colon, the tumor is T4b because it grows on another loop, not along the gastrointestinal route. The tumor also involves the serosal layer.

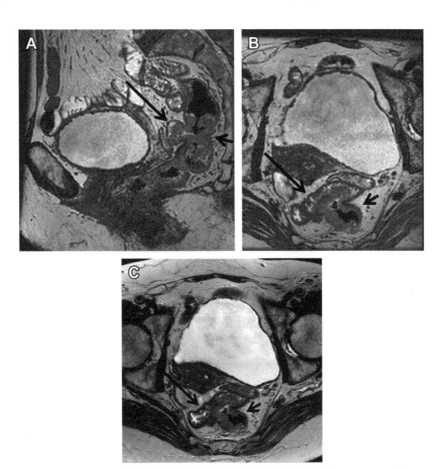

Fig. 12. (A) Sagittal 3D T2-weighted image of a patient with rectal cancer (*short arrow*) showing the tumor growing into a small bowel loop (*long arrow*). Reformatted axial (B) and true 2D axial (C) images show the same findings. Note the absence of chemical shift artifacts on 3D images and more noise, especially in soft tissues, compared with 2D images. This tumor should be designated T4b with growth into the serosal layer of peritoneum and small bowel.

difficulties because imaging the curved pelvic floor can be challenging. Benign tumors can be easily mistaken for malignant ones (due to false apparent extramural tumor component), or malignant tumor can be overstaged owing to the tumors coming closer to the pelvic floor. Imaging after radiotherapy often leads to disappearance of the large intraluminal portion, and this can improve accuracy, because often the rectum is collapsed after treatment. If multiplanar sequences are not available, one could use the typical behavior of rectal cancer growth. Usually tumors grow outwards from their epicenter both on transectional plane and along the longitudinal plane, with two exceptions. Very large tumors can extend beyond the rectal wall at several locations. Moreover, biopsies from the lower edge of tumors can lead to local perforations, a complication rarely seen.

Serosal layer The latest versions of TNM classification classify colorectal cancer extending into the serosa separately from tumors growing into other neighboring organs, all being referred to as T4. With the latest TNM classification (TNM7), serosal involvement is classified as T4a while involvement of other organs with or without serosa is classified as T4b (**Figs. 16** and **17**). This classification represents a reversal of previous ones in which involvement of all organs was T4a, and involvement of serosal layer with or without neighboring organs was T4b. There are no studies looking specifically at the accuracy of MR imaging (or CT) for assessment of local involvement of serosa. The only study coming close is that by Shihab and colleagues,[9] who evaluated 9 patients with T4b (according to TNM5), 7 of whom were accurately staged by

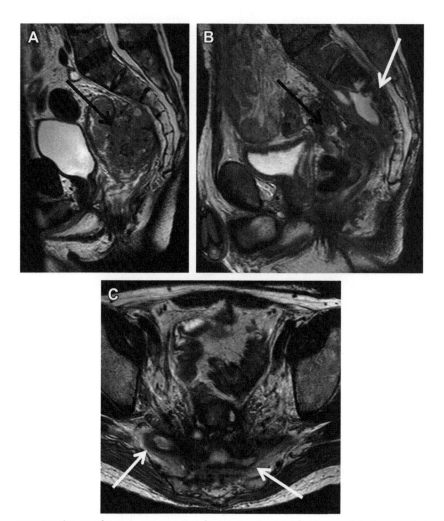

Fig. 13. An exceptional case of tumor progression during treatment. The tumor (*black arrows*) shown on the sagittal image (*A*) before treatment is extremely large and, despite growth into posterior mesorectal fascia, shows no growth into the sacral bone. The tumor shows marked size reduction after treatment (*B, C*); however, it has perforated and extended extensively via the foramina into the sacral bone (*white arrows*). It is nearly impossible to know whether these extensions contain tumor cells and whether the tumor is now T4 or not. Tumor perforations before treatment should be considered equal to tumor spread, however. Furthermore, perforation per se is no longer considered T4, even though the prognosis for tumor perforations remains poor.

MR imaging. In addition, 2 patients with T4b assessed by MR imaging did not show peritoneal pathologic involvement. This finding translates to 77.8% sensitivity and 97.5% specificity.

The following criteria may be used for involvement of serosa:

1. Tumor growing into another structure when and where that organ/structure is covered by peritoneum (definitive sign). This sign has less clinical significance today, owing to these tumors being classified as T4b according to TNM7
2. Tumor showing nodular growth through the peritoneal surface (definitive sign)

3. Abnormally placed peritoneal fluid in the absence of other reasons or simultaneous peritoneal carcinomatosis (suggestive signs)

Relation to muscularis propria layer
The basis for T1 to T3 staging according to TNM for colorectal cancer is the relation of tumor to the muscularis propria layer. Whereas larger T3 tumors are easy to distinguish, the distinction between T1, T2, and small T3 is elusive (**Fig. 18**). For this reason several approaches are suggested, such as using an endorectal probe, distension of the rectum, or use of endorectal or endoanal ultrasonography. Whereas endoscopic

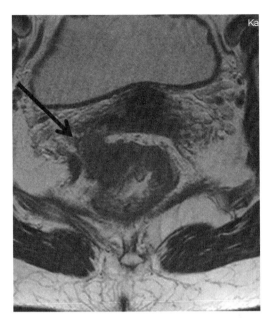

Fig. 14. Axial T2-weighted image showing rectal cancer growth into the posterior vaginal wall (*arrow*). Not all T4 tumors have the same significance, and therefore the extent of tumor growth should be provided. Posterior vaginal growth is considered one of more favorable forms of T4 tumors.

ultrasonography has reasonably high accuracy for discriminating T1 from the other T stages, differentiating T2 from small T3 is still not highly accurate. MR imaging with an endorectal probe is similar to endoscopic ultrasonography in terms of both accuracy and limitations.[14,15] Not reaching the location of interest is the most common problem. Endoluminal filling might help, especially in large polypoid lesions, by raising the intraluminal portion and making it float away from the rectal wall, thus preventing problems with staging (**Fig. 19**). Experience can overcome this problem otherwise. By tracing the origin of the tumor from the wall and ignoring where the tumor abuts the other sides, one can assign an accurate T stage. Usually a small amount of residual intraluminal fluid adjacent to the tumor may help to detect its location. Rectal filling might help in more flat lesions by stretching the rectal wall, and also differentiating "taenia recti" from tumor outgrowth. Rectum does not truly contain taeniae (unlike the colon). On the other hand, the taeniae of sigmoid colon do not finish abruptly at the rectosigmoid junction. Instead these taeniae disperse gradually, forming the longitudinal layer of muscularis propria. This transitional zone is 3 cm long, and because the rectum is folded ventrally at the rectosigmoid junction, these muscles can be seen bulging forward. Extreme

caution should be exercised in discerning these muscle bundles of lower SI from the intermediate SI of the tumor (**Fig. 20**).

Filling of the rectum, however, can have disadvantages. Opponents mention the problems of moving the rectal wall and its tumor falsely closer to MRF, and irritating the rectum, causing movement artifacts.[16] Rectal filling is therefore not recommended. The recommendation to carry out rectal filling is highly dependent on the policies of MDT (see the discussion on extramural tumor depth).

Extramural tumor depth in the mesorectal fat for T3 tumors

In some countries a modified TNM staging, based on the depth of T3 tumor growth into the perirectal/pericolic fat or extramural depth (EMD), is used for colorectal cancer. Up to 1 mm growth is considered T3a, 1 to 5 mm T3b, 5 to 15 mm T3c, and larger than 15 mm T3d. In some countries T3c-T3d rectal tumors are considered candidates for preoperative radiotherapy, whereas in others this distinction plays a minor role. In the latter countries all T3 tumors may receive preoperative radiotherapy. Such an approach makes the distinction between small T3 and T2 tumors much more important.

Two issues deserve extra attention, the first of which is the impact of imaging plane on EMD measurements (**Fig. 21**). The concept of EMD comes from pathologic reports initially. Pathologists have no possibility of reformatting their giant sections. Despite this, the MERCURY study was able to show that there was no discernible bias between MR imaging and histopathologic measurements.[17] Second, one can have an indefinite number of imaging planes perpendicular to a tube at any given point. Such complex geometry rules are usually forgotten and do not pose a problem in reality. Moreover, for extremely small or very large T3 tumors such meticulous measurements will not affect tumor classification. However, for those centers where treatment strategy is based on distinction between T3b and T3c, such millimeter precision becomes fundamental. Even MERCURY has shown that measurements between radiologists and pathologists differ roughly between minus 4 and plus 4 mm in 95% of cases. This disparity means that if a radiologist measures an EMD to be 4 mm, a pathologist might report any figure between 0 and 8 mm spanning from T2 to T3c. However, this is a reflection of arbitrarily chosen limits. The MDT must therefore be aware of such limitations. At many institutions this has led many MDTs to choose preoperative radiotherapy, even for larger T3b tumors.

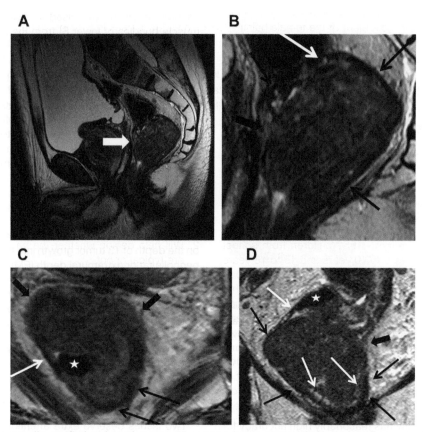

Fig. 15. A surgically verified polypoid tumor in rectum (*large thick white arrow*) shown on the sagittal T2-weighted image (*A*). Magnified view of sagittal (*B*), axial (*B*) and coronal view demonstrate a typical problem with such low tumors. Such a round tumor is often difficult to evaluate in several places because the muscularis propria becomes hazy (*large thick black arrows*), and suspicion of a T3 tumor (of if close to anterior organs or pelvic floor T4) is raised. There are several ways to solve this. One is to use rectal filling. Such an approach will make the tumor float and move away from the rectal wall. Another approach is use of ultrathin 3D imaging to avoid partial volume effect caused by nonperpendicular imaging planes. However, the radiologist then has to reformat the images. Experience can sometimes help. These polyps sometimes have pockets of fluid (*thin white arrows*) or gas (*white stars*). When these are seen close to the wall, there is no tumor breach through the wall. Also, the radiologist has to match different views on different images. *Black arrows* demonstrate intact rectal walls. One should look for the base of the polyp, usually denoted by more vessels. If there is an outgrowth, it is at the tumor base.

Another perhaps more serious issue is deciding what constitutes a tumor (**Fig. 22**). Mucin should be considered in the same way as tumors with nodular growth (see later discussion). However, tiny millimeter-thick strands can both be harboring tumor or be completely tumor free. Sometimes they can be difficult to differentiate from small vessels that seem to become more prominent at the area of the tumor. Whereas some studies have clearly shown that tiny tumor strands can have tumor cells, others have claimed that tiny strands are tumor free. The main difference in these studies might be the

inclusion of patients who have had short course of radiotherapy (5 Gy administered each day for 5 days) followed directly by surgery. It is conceivable that even short-term radiotherapy might render these tiny strands sterile. It is, therefore, once again crucial that the correct information is conveyed to members of the MDT.

Not all tiny strands are malignant. It is common to see a tiny strand reaching from the ventral aspect of rectum to anterior MRF/peritoneum. Such a strand is seen only in midline and is disproportionate to the tumor location and other tumor strands. Not infrequently the peritoneum is

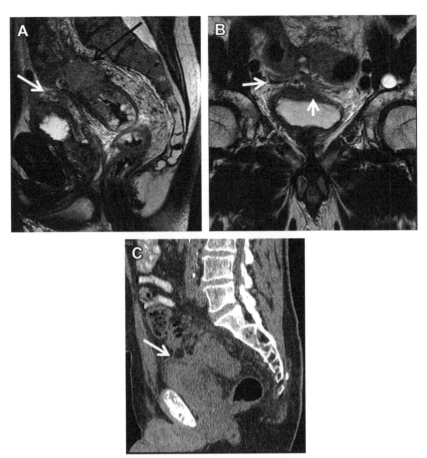

Fig. 16. A high rectal tumor (*black arrow*; definition on rectal vs sigmoid is based on rigid rectoscopy, not anatomy) growing into the peritoneal layer and urinary bladder.

reflected dorsally in the midline, simulating retraction caused by tumor. Such midline strands should not be considered malignant and are usually embryologic remnants. Therefore, the so-called seagull sign may not always reflect tumor growth.

Extramural venous invasion

Extramural venous tumor invasion (EMVI) is the most significant risk factor after T4 stage and involved CRM.[18] Assessment of EMVI is one of the shortcomings of pathologists, and perhaps there is more to be learned about assessment of EMVI (**Fig. 23**). Smith and colleagues[18] suggested a 5-point (0–4) scale system whereby obtaining 3 or more points corresponded to patients showing EMVI by the pathologist. Of note, they did not actually compare vessel for vessel. In fact the vessels called for EMVI assessment by the radiologists and pathologists might not even be the same.

In many centers EMVI is evaluated, although not usually classified by a score as in the MERCURY

study, keeping in mind that vessels involved with EMVI may not be close to the tumor itself.

The clinical significance of EMVI in all cases, and especially after treatment, is debatable. While EMVI has been shown to be related to relapse-free survival, the question is whether it plays a role if the patient already is manifesting metastatic disease. Also the significance of remaining radiologic EMVI after (chemo-)radiotherapy and before surgery can be questioned, as at the time of writing there is no impact on further treatment decision at restaging. Nonetheless, persistent EMVI after neoadjuvant therapy and long before surgery might necessitate more aggressive treatment.

Mucin

Mucin production by a tumor is a feature of adenocarcinomas. Mucin production is an interesting concept because its presence denotes worse prognosis. However, development of mucin during and after treatment can imply a favorable

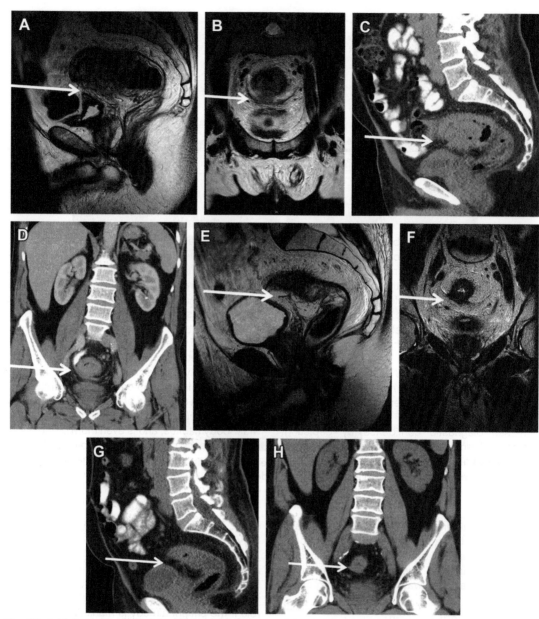

Fig. 17. A high rectal tumor (*arrow*) shown before (*A–D*) and after preoperative chemoradiotherapy (*E–H*). Both CT (*C, D*) and MR imaging (*A, B*) show tumor extension to peritoneum covering the urinary bladder. After chemoradiotherapy, however, only sagittal MR imaging (*E*) gives us to the clue to the final histopathologic result, namely that the tumor has regressed from the peritoneum and only fibrosis was seen reaching peritoneum.

response. Mucin pools are different from necrosis, the latter being more commonly associated with other tumor types such as SCC. Necrosis is due to reduced vascular supply whereas mucin reflects tumor differentiation grade. In radiology, necrosis is usually seen as a central fluid density on CT and fluid SI on MR imaging, surrounded by vascularized tumor tissue (**Fig. 24**). This feature is due to deficiency of blood supply for tissue demand. Mucin, on the other hand, can extend all the way to the periphery of tissue, hence the term mucin pool. Mucin pool is surrounded by a pseudocapsule. Whereas tumors with a soft-tissue component might abut adjacent organs

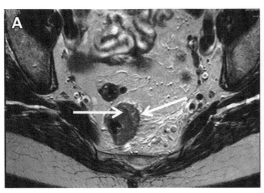
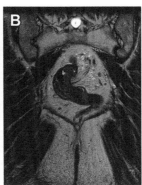
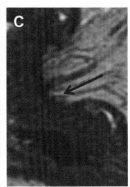

Fig. 18. A high rectal tumor. The axial scan (*A*) shows 2 muscular walls (*white arrows*) to the left side of the rectum. The coronal image (*B*) provides the explanation, which is the shape of rectum to the left. The prominent vessel (*black arrow in C*) entering shows why the bulk of the tumor is sometimes referred to the arrow sign. Magnification (*C*) shows the area where the tumor penetrates through the muscular wall. The tumor was shown to be a T3a tumor after surgery.

without invading them, it seems prudent to assume that all organs coming into contact with the pseudocapsule of mucin-producing tumors are compromised. Untreated mucin pools have been cultured and have shown potential for tumor growth (**Fig. 25**).[19]

Mucin can also act as a confounding factor in assessment by diffusion-weighted (DW) imaging, especially after treatment evaluation. Mucin behaves in the same way as fluid and necrosis, and usually has high SI on DW imaging. Apparent diffusion coefficient (ADC) values from mucin tumors are unreliable. However, the change in SI of tumors on DW imaging sometimes may reflect changes in mucin content, which is concordant with tumor response.

Lymph node staging

The Achilles heel of MR imaging (and pathology) in rectal cancer is nodal staging. N-staging is based on the number of malignant lymph nodes (and unofficially the ratio of malignant to all found nodes). The first studies on nodal staging therefore correlated N stages of radiology with stages of pathology. This policy changed after the work of some pioneers, and now most studies match lymph nodes. Although this probably has changed the view of how studies are conducted, clinicians still wish to know the N stage. TNM version 7 has an even more complex approach. It states that mesorectal tumor deposits are to be considered N1c in the absence of any other malignant lymph nodes. Considering the limited accuracy of radiologic N staging, the value of radiologic N staging, especially N0 or N1, has come under scrutiny. Several large studies put the same weight on radiologic N0 and N1 stages. This approach has much merit, as prognosis for N1 patients is closer to N0 than to N2.

Some nodal locations deserve extra attention.[10] The issue of nodes close to MRF has already been covered in the section regarding MRF. Nodes close to the area of vessel pedicle ligature close to the origin inferior mesenteric arteries should be especially scrutinized (**Fig. 26**). However, this is seldom a problem. Nodes outside the MRF may be located retroperitoneally in the prevertebral space, or extraperitoneally in the lateral

Fig. 19. Axial image of a patient with 2 tumors, a benign rectal polyp (*black arrow*) and a T3 tumor (*black arrow*). The distension by fluid inside the rectum facilitates T3 assessment and also causes the polyp to float.

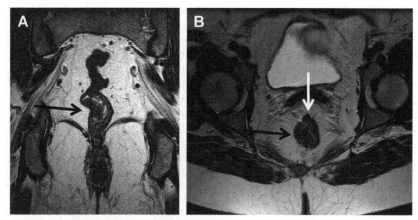

Fig. 20. A tumor in the middle of the rectum (*black arrows*) seen on coronal (*A*) and axial (*B*) images. Note the prominent muscle bundle (*white arrow*) at the level of upper part of the vagina. Here the thick muscle bundle provides a clear band of low SI. Had the muscle fibers been less prominent and the tumor located ventrally, the partial volume effect might have simulated tumor outgrowth.

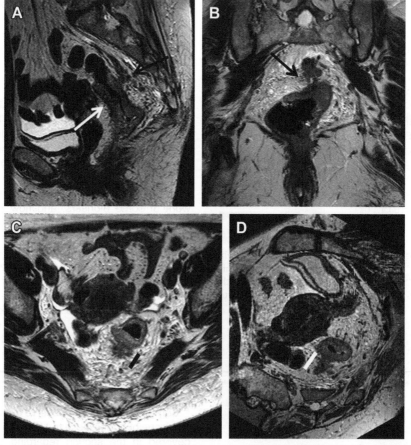

Fig. 21. Problem with the measurement of extramural tumor depth (EMD). Sagittal image (*A*) shows a straight-forward case of a tumor (*black arrow*) for EMD measurements. The coronal image (*B*), however, reveals that the rectum is actually turning in a right to left direction as it moves up. Imaging in the plane (*C*) perpendicular to rectum based on the sagittal plane shows the EMD (*black bar*). However, a slightly tilted image (*D*) derived from a 3D image with the same magnification as C shows a slightly larger EMD (*white bar*). Compare the cross sections of rectal lumen on C and D; on image D the rectum appears to be more circular, therefore the imaging plane must be closer to truly perpendicular.

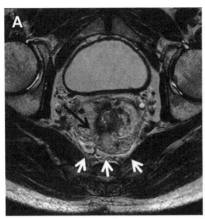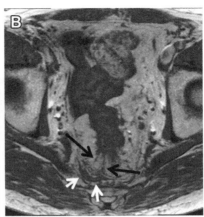

Fig. 22. A rectal cancer with tiny strands (*black arrows*) that contain tumor. Both T2-weighted (*A*) and T1-weighted imaging (*B*) show the tiny strands against the fat background of mesorectal fat. Intermediate SI similar to that of the tumor on T2-weighted imaging helps further. In this case the tiny tumor strands reach the dorsal mesorectal fascia to the right and lift it off the presacral fascia, creating a space filled with fluid (*small white arrows*). This fluid has high signal on T2-weighted imaging (*A*) and may completely be missed, while on T1-weighted imaging it is seen more clearly.

spaces of the pelvis, so-called extramesorectal nodes (**Fig. 27**). Theoretically the presence of these nodal groups in rectal cancer would suggest distant metastatic disease; however, calling each lateral pelvic node malignant might be an exaggeration. These nodes are extremely rare as the cause of recurrent disease.[20] Furthermore, involvement of these nodes is seldom an independent prognostic risk factor.

Various different criteria have been used for nodal assessment.[21] Heterogeneous lymph nodes are much more often malignant than are homogenous nodes. Sometimes the heterogeneous feature is appreciated better on CT than on MR imaging. Mucin and amorphous calcifications are reliable signs of malignancy on both CT and MR imaging; however, mucin is more easily appreciated on MR imaging compared with CT, whereas for calcification the opposite is true. Of interest, mucin and calcifications are not infrequently coexistent. Mucin might be the most specific sign of malignancy. Presence of fatty hilum is usually considered a predictive sign of benignity, especially in larger nodes.

Nodal size has been used extensively as a criterion for diagnosing malignancy in earlier studies (**Fig. 28**). However, most malignant mesorectal nodes are smaller than 5 mm. A mesorectal node larger than 1 to 2 cm in the longest short diameter is likely to be malignant, and no visible nodes on MR imaging is likely to indicate N0 status.

A round node is more likely than an elliptical node to be malignant. One should remember, however, that nodes are 3-dimensional. Benign nodes are often round in the plane perpendicular to the vessels they are adjacent to. Irregular, non-smooth borders should raise suspicions of malignancy.

The role of DW imaging and gadolinium contrast has not been consolidated. There is currently no contrast agent commercially available for lymph node staging.

Good, bad, and ugly
The concept of good, bad, and ugly is based on tumor features that predict prognosis. It is assumed that "good-looking" tumors need the least intensive treatment while "ugly tumors" need the most intensive treatment. Though true to large extent, this assumes that only 3 options are available. It is noteworthy that just as for the concept of good, bad, and ugly, any other attempt to classify rectal cancer is subjective. It might be best to report what is seen on the images rather than to try categorizing the findings into certain groups.

For most centers, T1N0 tumors without any adverse prognostic indicators are considered good tumors. T4 or tumors with threatened/involved MRF are considered ugly. EMVI and/or T3c-T3d usually are considered as bad or ugly. T3a-T3b and N1-N2 stages are somewhat "wild card," moving between all 3 groups depending on the local policy of the MDT.[22] Mucin and low location usually do not play any direct role in such classification. Tumor perforation was previously considered a sign of T4 disease. However, it is unclear whether perforated tumors should be regarded as T4 nowadays.

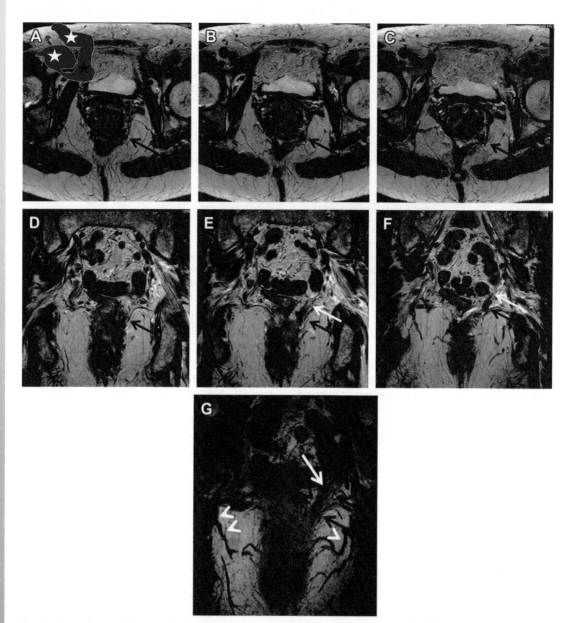

Fig. 23. Large low rectal tumor shown on 3 consecutive axial (*A–C*) and coronal (*D–F*) T2-weighted images. The outline of the tumor is shown as a gray inset on image *A*. Note that the tumor is not totally circumferential, and the outer bulges (shows by *white stars*) are not as important as the belly/center (*black star*) of the tumor. The tumor outgrowth is usually at this latter area (*black arrows*). Coronal images depict this tumor outgrowth reaching the middle rectal vein (*white arrows*). (*G*) A minimum-intensity projection made from thin (1 mm) original sagittal 3D T2-weighted images. Note the homogeneous low signal of the vessels (*white arrowheads*). It is easier to appreciate the perivascular growth of the tumor (*black arrows*) engulfing the middle rectal vein (*white arrow*) and the disruption of the vessel (*black arrowhead*), where there is also intravascular growth.

Evaluation of Preoperative Response

The use of MR imaging is clearly justified when the clinical situation demands such interim MR imaging before final surgery, for instance in cases of suspicion of tumor perforation or progression during or after treatment. Tumor progression, however, is exceptional. Routine use of MR imaging during or after preoperative radiotherapy should therefore be reserved for research

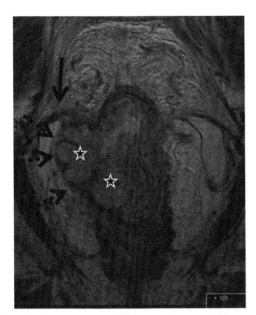

Fig. 24. A large low rectal tumor. The mucin component (*stars*) is a sign of the tumor being an adenocarcinoma and not a squamous cell carcinoma, despite being mainly situated under the pelvic floor (*solid black arrow*). With lower echo time, such as the one on this image, the mucin and fat have virtually the same SI. The boundaries of the mucin or pseudocapsule (*dotted arrows*) should not be mistaken for stretched sphincter muscle. This tumor is a T4, owing to involvement of the pelvic floor, and also has grown into the ischioanal fat.

between fibrosis with and without small tumor remnant. The trend is to defer from surgery in the very well responding patients, especially in those who have endoscopic and MR signs of complete tumor regression. Although complete disappearance of lymph nodes, especially small ones, makes assessment of MR imaging after chemoradiotherapy much easier, remaining lymph nodes are still elusive to certain diagnoses.

DW imaging, volumetry, and imaging with nonspecific contrast agents with or without perfusion have also been used for evaluating tumor response (**Fig. 29**).[14,26–28] A decrease in SI and/or the size of the area with high SI on DW imaging have been shown to correlate with response rate; however, the results have been inconsistent. ADC before or after, and ADC change have all been addressed, with some studies claiming promise and others not.

Initial tumor volume, residual tumor volume, and change in tumor volume correlate with response to varying degrees.

Both CT and MR perfusion studies have provided clues that tumor response can be measured on postcontrast imaging. These results have been very much like those of ^{18}F-fluorodeoxyglucose positron emission tomography (FDG-PET) showing that decreasing metabolic activity is associated with favorable response.[29] All of the aforementioned are more complex to apply during everyday routine.[30]

purposes or centers that act on information from new MR imaging. Treatment modification might be in the form of:

1. Therapy intensification (in stable disease) or
2. Removal of less tissue/organ than originally planned (in cases with marked tumor regression)

There is as yet not enough information to recommend therapy intensification based on interim MR imaging results, and thus most MR imaging is performed to limit the extent of originally planned surgery. The most reliable signs have been the appearance of completely clean fatty interface between tumor and the nearby organ in question. Tiny strands are also considered likely to be tumor free after treatment.[23–25]

Another scenario is complete disappearance of all tumor manifestations, including mesorectal lymph nodes on both T2-weighted and DW imaging. Very low SI of the rectal wall at the site of tumor is often seen, which suggests fibrosis. MR imaging, however, cannot differentiate

Local Recurrence

The indication for imaging for local recurrence usually arises when, after treatment and during surveillance, the patient develops symptoms or the carcinoembryonic antigen (CEA) levels increase. CT and FDG-PET/CT are both good methods for finding and confirming local recurrence (**Fig. 30**). These methods also help find out if the disease is present at other locations. Conditions such as diverticulitis can cause a slight increase in CEA, but high levels of CEA are often associated with tumor recurrence, either locally or distant. If curative resection of a proven local recurrence is considered, imaging can be helpful in planning surgery. In this instance MR imaging is the most accurate modality.[31] T2-weighted turbo spin-echo imaging probably is the best modality, although both DW imaging and/or postcontrast imaging might improve confidence in finding other tumor manifestations or perhaps even the extent of the already known tumor.

To increase detection, DW imaging before and after gadolinium and T2-weighted imaging is

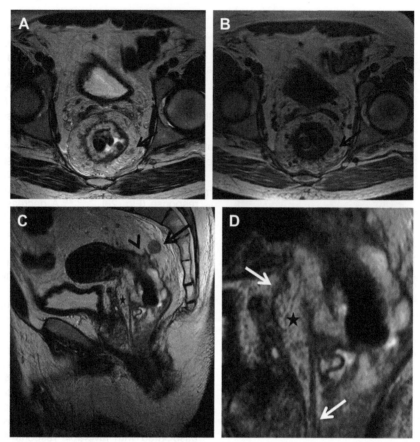

Fig. 25. A large mucin-producing tumor in mid rectum. (*A*) Axial T2-weighted image shows the tumor (*arrow*). However, it can be difficult sometimes to detect the extent of the tumor. A T1-weighted image (*B*) can help detect lymph nodes (*arrow*), which also shows that the high SI of the nodes is not due to fat but mucin. T1-weighted images, however, cannot help differentiate tumor from edema. (*C*) Sagittal image of the same patient shows another enlarged node (*arrow*), extramural venous invasion (*arrowhead*), and the anterior extent of the tumor. (*D*) A zoomed-in image shows the mucin extension (*star*) between the white arrows filling up the space between rectum and the prostate and seminal vesicles.

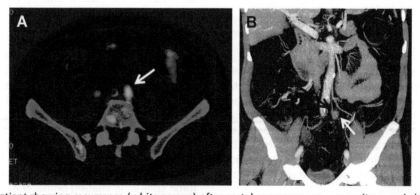

Fig. 26. A patient showing recurrence (*white arrows*) after rectal cancer surgery on positron emission tomography (PET) combined with CT (*A*). The resolution of PET is not high enough to elucidate whether the node is retroperitoneal (and thus a sign of spread disease) or a mesorectal node left behind (where extended surgery might be curative). The maximum-intensity projection CT of the abdomen and pelvis (*B*) show that the tumor is close to the long remaining superior rectal vessel (*black arrow*), and therefore most probably is the result of inadequate surgery. This node could not be seen on original MR imaging (too high), and on original CT images no corresponding node could be found.

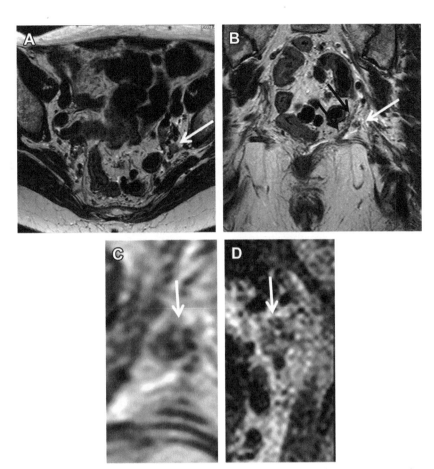

Fig. 27. Axial (*A*) and coronal (*B*) T2-weighted images from the same patient shown in **Fig. 23**. The axial image is higher and the coronal image more dorsally located than the ones shown in **Fig. 23**. Both images show a somewhat enlarged node in the internal iliac group (*white arrows*). The black arrows show tumor growth along the mesorectal fascia. Image *C* is the magnification of image *B* concerning the node in question while image *D* is a near coronal image reformatted from original sagittal 3D T2-weighted images. The heterogeneity of the node and somewhat irregular border could be consistent with malignancy. The patient was imaged in December 2008, received preoperative radiotherapy, and the node virtually disappeared on follow-up images (not shown). The patient has not shown any signs of pelvic recurrence up until October 2012.

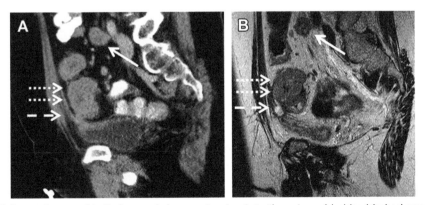

Fig. 28. A high rectal cancer (*dotted arrows*) shows extension into the urinary bladder (*dashed arrow*). Both CT (*A*) and MR imaging (*B*) show an enlarged lymph node (*white solid arrows*). Both modalities show irregular contours and heterogeneity.

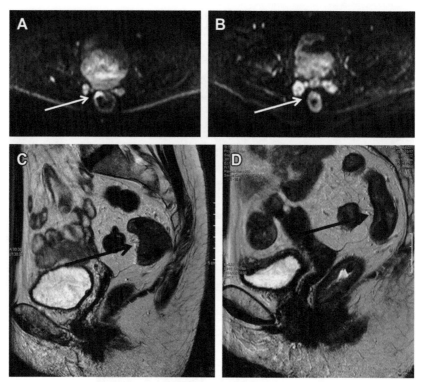

Fig. 29. A patient with rectal cancer (*white arrows*) located anteriorly and somewhat to the right on image before treatment (*A*), and the corresponding site after preoperative radiotherapy (*B*). The area with highest signal on diffusion-weighted imaging corresponded to the location of the tumor, and after treatment this is normalized. Sagittal T2-weighted images before (*C*) and after (*D*) treatment corroborate the disappearance of the tumor (*black arrows*).

recommended. Knowledge of the usual location of local recurrence improves the performance in detecting a recurrence. Most recurrences are anastomotic and are found by the surgeon.[32] Other recurrences may be found in remaining mesorectal fat in patients treated with low anterior resection, lateral pelvic nodes, mesorectal nodes, and presacrally. Presacral recurrence can be sometimes difficult to distinguish from normal changes after previous radiotherapy. Asymmetric appearance, heterogeneous and/or marked contrast enhancement, progressive enlargement over time, and invasive behavior point to malignancy, rather than postoperative findings. Review of the first postoperative images is highly recommended because recurrences can grow slowly, and comparison with only the most recent previous examination may easily overlook a local recurrence. Sometimes recurrence of rectal cancer manifests by metastasis to pelvic organs, most notably ovaries and peritoneal implants, which are not true "local" recurrences.

The most difficult scenario occurs when an abscess is seen presacrally. CEA levels and FDG-PET/CT do not help. Leakage is often the cause of abscess, and patients with postoperative leaks have a higher incidence of local recurrence. Biopsies are difficult and, not infrequently, inconclusive. Imaging can offer limited help unless overt signs of invasive disease that point to malignancy are seen. Presence of prominent lymph nodes should be considered as highly suggestive of malignancy rather than a simple abscess.

Not infrequently the tumor invades the sacrum or presacral space. Under these conditions 2 questions are most pertinent. First one needs to find out if the sacrum is resectable. Most surgeons remove the sacrum and coccyx up to the level of S2; however, tumor involving S1 or higher are not considered resectable. Furthermore, tumors invading the presacral space or sacrum have direct access to the retroperitoneal space. In this case retroperitoneal lymph nodes should be assessed carefully, and for this goal FDG-PET/CT

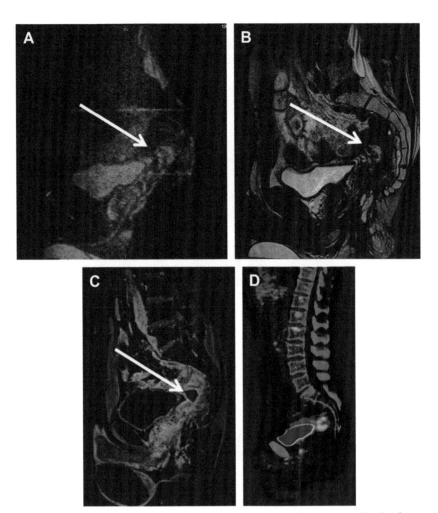

Fig. 30. Sagittal images from an individual imaged at another center with increasing levels of carcinoembryonic antigen. Diffusion-weighted imaging (*A*), sagittal T2-weighted images (*B*), and contrast-enhanced T1-weighted images (*C*) can have varying degrees of success demonstrating local recurrence (*white arrows*). In this particular case and most other cases, contrast-enhanced images provide the best clue. PET/CT (*D*) is often used and can often help.

and, more importantly, comparison with older images might prove helpful. However, enlarged reactive lymph nodes with slightly increased FDG uptake always pose a problem.

MR IMAGING OF ANAL CANCER

Because anal cancer (or more correctly SCC of the anorectal region [**Fig. 31**]) is less common, it seems prudent that tertiary centers should become the main provider of diagnosis and staging. The role of MR imaging in anal cancer is mostly in staging of the disease or its recurrence. However, because radiotherapy achieves high cure rates in most cases, in addition to the simpler nature of anal cancer, MR imaging of anal cancer

is much easier to evaluate than imaging of rectal cancer.[32–35]

T Staging

T staging in anal cancer is mainly conducted by measuring the tumor in its longest diameter (**Figs. 32** and **33**). One has to remember that this longest diameter is often not axial.

Stage T4, however, is somewhat tricky. Depending on where the bulk of the tumor is located, the definition of neighboring organs varies. The European Society of Medical Oncology (ESMO) answered some of these questions in 2010. The authors acknowledge the following organs that do not affect T4 staging, based on ESMO

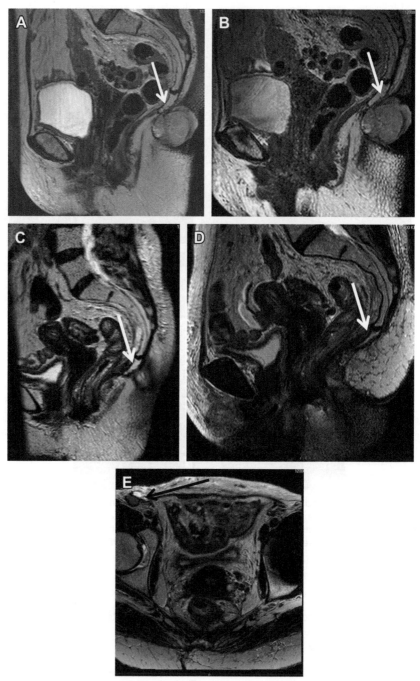

Fig. 31. A squamous cell cancer of perianal region that is classified and treated as anal cancer shown on 2D (*A*) and 3D (*B*) sagittal T2-weighted images. The dorsal cortical bone of the coccyx seems to be eroded on the thinner slice, with suspicion of tumor growth (*white arrow*). Imaging after treatment (*C*) with 1.5 T shows considerable shrinkage in tumor size, but still with the defect in the cortical bone. The patient undergoes surgery and the surgeon notices no growth into the bone. The distance to resection margin is 1 to 2 mm of loose fat. Imaging after surgery (*D*, *E*) reveals no tumor rests locally, but recurrence in the form of an inguinal node (*black arrow*).

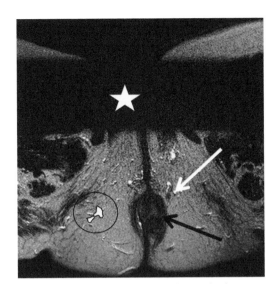

Fig. 32. Small T1 anal cancer (*black arrow*). The tumor is T1 because its largest diameter is less than 2 cm. The outlines of the tumors are shown separately as an inset inside the circle. Note the lymph node in the ischioanal fossa (*white arrow*). If malignant these nodes are not addressed by TNM staging. Note also the large saturation band (*star*) that obscures any assessment of inguinal lymph nodes.

guidelines, official TNM handbooks, and their own experience:

1. The external and/or internal sphincter muscles for all types of anal cancer
2. Rectal wall for all types of anal cancer
3. Puborectalis muscle for all tumors
4. Vestibule for tumors originating from anal margin (Fig. 34)

5. Continuous involvement of levator ani muscle for tumors of the anal canal

Once again, correct conveyance of information to members of the MDT rather than strict classification is desirable.

N and M Staging

Nodal staging of anal cancer, in contrast to that of other adenocarcinomas of the gastrointestinal tract such as the rectum, is based on the involvement lymph node stations rather than the number of lymph nodes involved (Figs. 35 and 36). ESMO recommends different N staging for cancer of the anal margin and anal canal. All lymph nodes behind the external iliac vessels are considered to belong to the obturator fossa and thus are part of the internal iliac group. Nodes along external and common iliac vessels are considered as distant spread. The most common distant metastases at the time of initial staging are located in the pelvis. A particular group easily overlooked is nodes just below the aortic bifurcation. These nodes are missed on CT by inexperienced radiologists because they appear just under the aorta on axial sections.[36,37] MR radiologists can also easily miss these nodes, partially because the focus of imaging is on the anal canal and not the whole pelvis (see below).

The following criteria for the diagnosis of lymph node metastases in patients with anal cancer are suggested:

1. Markedly enlarged nodes based on their largest short-axis diameter (≥ 1 cm mesorectal, ≥ 1.6 cm for internal iliac, and ≥ 2 cm for all other nodes including inguinal nodes)

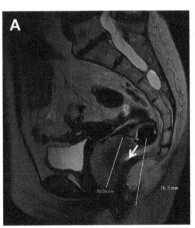
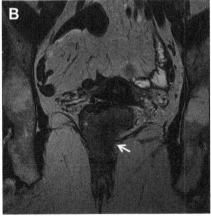

Fig. 33. A large squamous cell cancer (*arrow*) located mainly above the anal canal shown on sagittal (*A*) and coronal (*B*) views. The tumor length measured is more than 5 cm and therefore is at least T3. However, the tumor involves the levator ani muscle and therefore can be classified as T4.

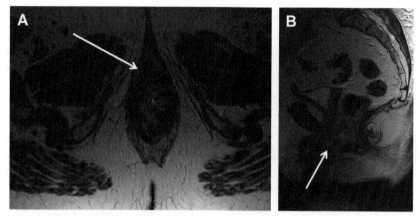

Fig. 34. Axial (*A*) and sagittal (*B*) images of an anal cancer involving the lower ends of the vagina and urethra (*white arrows*). The tumor is mainly from the anal canal and therefore a T4.

2. Necrosis in nodes or clear heterogeneity
3. Stronger enhancement of small nodes than the tumor itself

The imaging protocol should cover the inguinal areas and higher nodal stations adequately. The same meticulous imaging of the primary tumor as for rectal cancer is not necessary. Whereas contrast enhancement is not used for MR imaging of rectal cancer, it is probably beneficial for anal cancer (similarly to other SCCs of the pelvis). Finally, the role of DW imaging in anal cancer has yet to be determined,

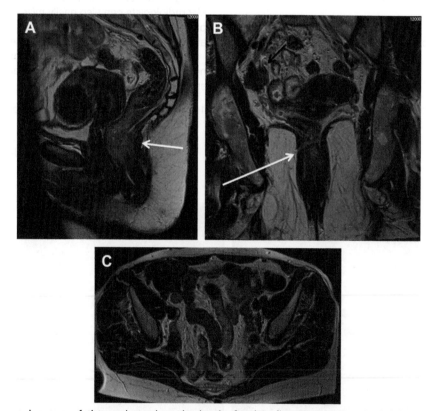

Fig. 35. An anal cancer of the anal canal at the level of pelvic floor seen on sagittal (*A*) and coronal (*B*) T2-weighted images. The tumor is between 2 and 5 cm and could be classified as T2. It grows into the puborectal muscle (*white arrows*), which does not change the classification. Note also the bilateral internal iliac node metastases (*black arrows*) seen on the coronal (*B*) and axial images. The tumor is thus N3.

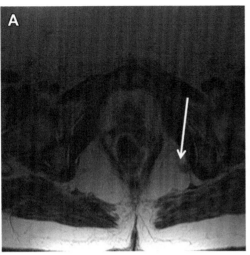
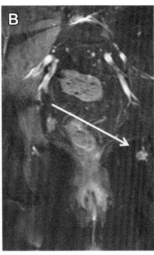

Fig. 36. (*A, B*) A patient with anal cancer (not shown) and unusual nodular metastasis close to internal obturator muscle (*arrows*). The metastasis is shown clearly on contrast-enhanced images. This case also illustrates the limitations of TNM staging system. Is this a lymph node or a muscular metastasis? If a lymph node, is it a local or a distant lymph node? The most important issue is to convey the message as well as limitations to the clinicians at the MDT meeting.

and might prove to be different from the role of DW imaging in rectal cancer.

REFERENCES

1. Glynne-Jones R, Northover JM, Cervantes A. Anal cancer: ESMO clinical practice guidelines for diagnosis, treatment and follow-up. Ann Oncol 2010; 21(Suppl 5):v87–92.
2. Birgisson H, Talbäck M, Gunnarsson U, et al. Improved survival in cancer of the colon and rectum in Sweden. Eur J Surg Oncol 2005;31(8):845–53.
3. den Dulk M, Krijnen P, Marijnen CA, et al. Improved overall survival for patients with rectal cancer since 1990: the effects of TME surgery and pre-operative radiotherapy. Eur J Cancer 2008;44(12):1710–6.
4. Lemmens V, van Steenbergen L, Janssen-Heijnen M, et al. Trends in colorectal cancer in the south of the Netherlands 1975-2007: rectal cancer survival levels with colon cancer survival. Acta Oncol 2010;49(6):784–96.
5. Oistämö E, Hjern F, Blomqvist L, et al. Cancer and diverticulitis of the sigmoid colon. Differentiation with computed tomography versus magnetic resonance imaging: preliminary experiences. Acta Radiol 2013;54(3):237–41.
6. Heald RJ, Ryall RD. Recurrence and survival after total mesorectal excision for rectal cancer. Lancet 1986;1:1479–82.
7. Beets-Tan RG, Beets GL, Vliegen RF, et al. Accuracy of magnetic resonance imaging in prediction of tumour-free resection margin in rectal cancer surgery. Lancet 2001;357(9255):497–504.
8. Beets-Tan RG, Lambregts DM, Maas M, et al. Magnetic resonance imaging for the clinical management of rectal cancer patients: recommendations from the 2012 European Society of Gastrointestinal and Abdominal Radiology (ESGAR) consensus meeting. Eur Radiol 2013. http://dx.doi.org/10.1007/s00330-013-2864-4.
9. Shihab OC, Quirke P, Heald RJ, et al. Magnetic resonance imaging-detected lymph nodes close to the mesorectal fascia are rarely a cause of margin involvement after total mesorectal excision. Br J Surg 2010;97(9):1431–6.
10. Torkzad MR, Påhlman L, Glimelius B. Magnetic resonance imaging (MRI) in rectal cancer: a comprehensive review. Insights Imaging 2010;1(4):245–67.
11. Shihab OC, Heald RJ, Rullier E, et al. Defining the surgical planes on MRI improves surgery for cancer of the low rectum. Lancet Oncol 2009;10(12):1207–11.
12. Gowdra Halappa V, Corona Villalobos CP, Bonekamp S, et al. Rectal imaging: part 1, High-resolution MRI of carcinoma of the rectum at 3 T. AJR Am J Roentgenol 2012;199(1):W35–42.
13. Fütterer JJ, Yakar D, Strijk SP, et al. Preoperative 3T MR imaging of rectal cancer: local staging accuracy using a two-dimensional and three-dimensional T2-weighted turbo spin echo sequence. Eur J Radiol 2008;65(1):66–71.
14. Kim SH, Lee JM, Hong SH, et al. Locally advanced rectal cancer: added value of diffusion-weighted MR imaging in the evaluation of tumor response to neoadjuvant chemo- and radiation therapy. Radiology 2009;253(1):116–25.

15. Dinter DJ, Hofheinz RD, Hartel M, et al. Preoperative staging of rectal tumors: comparison of endorectal ultrasound, hydro-CT, and high-resolution endorectal MRI. Onkologie 2008;31(5):230–5.

16. Slater A, Halligan S, Taylor SA, et al. Distance between the rectal wall and mesorectal fascia measured by MRI: effect of rectal distension and implications for preoperative prediction of a tumour-free circumferential resection margin. Clin Radiol 2006;61(1):65–70.

17. MERCURY Study Group. Extramural depth of tumor invasion at thin-section MR in patients with rectal cancer: results of the MERCURY study. Radiology 2007;243(1):132–9.

18. Smith NJ, Shihab O, Arnaout A, et al. MRI for detection of extramural vascular invasion in rectal cancer. AJR Am J Roentgenol 2008;191(5):1517–22.

19. Yantiss RK, Shia J, Klimstra DS, et al. Prognostic significance of localized extra-appendiceal mucin deposition in appendiceal mucinous neoplasms. Am J Surg Pathol 2009;33(2):248–55.

20. Syk E, Torkzad MR, Blomqvist L, et al. Radiological findings do not support lateral residual tumour as a major cause of local recurrence of rectal cancer. Br J Surg 2006;93(1):113–9.

21. Matsuoka H, Nakamura A, Masaki T, et al. Optimal diagnostic criteria for lateral pelvic lymph node metastasis in rectal carcinoma. Anticancer Res 2007;27(5B):3529–33.

22. Guillem JG, Díaz-González JA, Minsky BD, et al. cT3N0 rectal cancer: potential overtreatment with preoperative chemoradiotherapy is warranted. J Clin Oncol 2008;26(3):368–73.

23. Vliegen RF, Beets GL, Lammering G, et al. Mesorectal fascia invasion after neoadjuvant chemotherapy and radiation therapy for locally advanced rectal cancer: accuracy of MR imaging for prediction. Radiology 2008;246(2):454–62.

24. Torkzad MR, Suzuki C, Tanaka S, et al. Morphological assessment of the interface between tumor and neighboring tissues, by magnetic resonance imaging, before and after radiotherapy in patients with locally advanced rectal cancer. Acta Radiol 2008;49(10):1099–103.

25. Lahaye MJ, Beets GL, Engelen SM, et al. Locally advanced rectal cancer: MR imaging for restaging after neoadjuvant radiation therapy with concomitant chemotherapy. Part II. What are the criteria to predict involved lymph nodes? Radiology 2009;252(1):81–91.

26. Dresen RC, Beets GL, Rutten HJ, et al. Locally advanced rectal cancer: MR imaging for restaging after neoadjuvant radiation therapy with concomitant chemotherapy. Part I. Are we able to predict tumor confined to the rectal wall? Radiology 2009;252(1):71–80.

27. Torkzad M, Lindholm J, Martling A, et al. Retrospective measurement of different size parameters of non-radiated rectal cancer on MR images and pathology slides and their comparison. Eur Radiol 2003;13(10):2271–7.

28. Torkzad MR, Lindholm J, Martling A, et al. MRI after preoperative radiotherapy for rectal cancer; correlation with histopathology and the role of volumetry. Eur Radiol 2007;17(6):1566–73.

29. Rosenberg R, Herrmann K, Gertler R, et al. The predictive value of metabolic response to preoperative radiochemotherapy in locally advanced rectal cancer measured by PET/CT. Int J Colorectal Dis 2009;24(2):191–200.

30. Smith JA, Wild AT, Singhi A, et al. Clinicopathologic comparison of high-dose-rate endorectal brachytherapy versus conventional chemoradiotherapy in the neoadjuvant setting for resectable stages II and III low rectal cancer. Int J Surg Oncol 2012;2012:406568.

31. Messiou C, Chalmers AG, Boyle K, et al. Pre-operative MR assessment of recurrent rectal cancer. Br J Radiol 2008;81(966):468–73.

32. Syk E, Torkzad MR, Blomqvist L, et al. Local recurrence in rectal cancer: anatomic localization and effect on radiation target. Int J Radiat Oncol Biol Phys 2008;72(3):658–64.

33. Kochhar R, Plumb AA, Carrington BM, et al. Imaging of anal carcinoma. AJR Am J Roentgenol 2012;199:W335–44.

34. Roach SC, Hulse PA, Moulding FJ, et al. Magnetic resonance imaging of anal cancer. Clin Radiol 2005;60:1111–9.

35. Tonolini M, Bianco R. MRI and CT of anal carcinoma: a pictorial review. Insights Imaging 2013;4(1):53–62.

36. Wells IT, Fox BM. PET/CT in anal cancer - is it worth doing? Clin Radiol 2012;67(6):535–40.

37. Bhuva NJ, Glynne-Jones R, Sonoda L, et al. To PET or not to PET? That is the question. Staging in anal cancer. Ann Oncol 2012;23(8):2078–82.

Magnetic Resonance Imaging of Perianal Fistulas

Dirk Vanbeckevoort, MD[a,*], Didier Bielen, MD, PhD[a,b], Ragna Vanslembrouck, MD[a], Gert Van Assche, MD, PhD[c,d]

KEYWORDS

- Fistula • MR imaging • Perianal • Crohn disease

KEY POINTS

- MR imaging has been shown to accurately show the anatomy of the perianal region.
- Currently, MR imaging is also a reliable technique to assess the outcome of medical therapy using the anti-TNF agent infliximab in patients with Crohn disease with fistula-in-ano occurring during the first year of follow-up.
- Another important advantage of MR imaging is the multiplanar assessment. However, imaging planes must be correctly aligned to the anal canal.
- Despite the closure of draining external orifices after infliximab therapy, fistula tracks persist with varying degrees of residual inflammation, which may cause recurrent fistulas and pelvic abscesses.

INTRODUCTION

Perianal fistulas are a major cause of morbidity. Fistulas are defined as an abnormal communication between 2 epithelium-lined surfaces. In the case of a perianal fistula, the connection is between the mucosal layer of the anal canal and the perianal skin.

Perianal fistulas predominantly affect young adults, especially men in their fourth decade.[1]

Treatment of perianal fistulizing disease is medical or surgical. Patients with Crohn disease are first treated with antibiotics, immunosuppressive agents, or anti–tumor necrosis factor (anti-TNF) antibodies. Fistulas not related to Crohn disease are usually treated with surgery.[2]

Recurrence after therapy is the most common problem. To avoid recurrence after medical or surgical therapy, detailed information must be obtained about the location of any fistula track and the affected pelvic structures. High-resolution magnetic resonance (MR) imaging allows precise assessment of the relationship of the fistula track to the pelvic floor structures, and identification of secondary fistulas or abscesses.

NORMAL ANAL CANAL ANATOMY

Underneath the mucosa, the anal canal consists of an internal layer of circular smooth muscle (the internal sphincter) and an outer striated muscle layer (the external sphincter). The 2 sphincters are separated by the intersphincteric space, which contains predominantly fat (**Fig. 1**). This space forms a natural plane of lower resistance in which fistulas can easily spread.[3] The external sphincter is surrounded by the fat-containing ischiorectal and ischioanal space.[2]

The internal sphincter is continuous with the circular smooth muscle of the rectum. It is responsible for 85% of the anal resting tone.[4] In most individuals, disruption of the sphincter will not cause loss of continence.[5]

Dr Didier Bielen is the 'joint first author' for this article.
The authors have nothing to disclose.
[a] Department of Radiology, University Hospitals Leuven, Herestraat 49, Leuven B-3000, Belgium; [b] Department of Imaging and Pathology, KU Leuven, Herestraat 49, Leuven 3000, Belgium; [c] Department of Gastroenterology, University Hospitals Leuven, Herestraat 49, Leuven 3000, Belgium; [d] Department of Clinical and Experimental Medicine, KU Leuven, Herestraat 49, Leuven 3000, Belgium
* Corresponding author.
E-mail address: dirk.vanbeckevoort@uzleuven.be

Magn Reson Imaging Clin N Am 22 (2014) 113–123
http://dx.doi.org/10.1016/j.mric.2013.07.008
1064-9689/14/$ – see front matter © 2014 Elsevier Inc. All rights reserved.

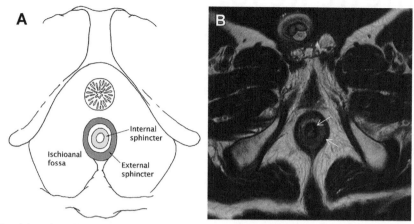

Fig. 1. Drawing (*A*) and axial T2-weighted MR image (*B*) show the normal anatomy of the perianal region (at the level of the mid-anal canal). *Arrows* indicate internal and external sphincter.

The external sphincter is continuous with the puborectal and levator ani muscles (**Fig. 2**). It contributes only 15% of the anal resting tone, but its strong voluntary contractions resist defecation. A disruption of the external sphincter can lead to incontinence.[5]

MR imaging has been shown to accurately show the anatomy of the perianal region. On axial T2-weighted images, the internal and external anal sphincter appear as circular structures with low signal intensity.

After intravenous administration of gadolinium, the internal and external sphincter can be easily distinguished on T1-weighted images by their different contrast enhancement. The internal sphincter muscle enhances to a higher degree than the external sphincter muscle (**Fig. 3**).[6,7]

CAUSE OF PERIANAL FISTULAS

In patients without Crohn disease, perianal fistulas usually arise from infected or obstructed intersphincteric anal glands (cryptogenic fistulas).[8] The anal glands lie at the level of the dentate line in the mid-anal canal and can penetrate the internal sphincter toward the intersphincteric plane (intersphincteric fistula). From this space, the infection may track down the intersphincteric plane to the skin. Alternatively, infection may pass both layers of the anal sphincter to enter the ischiorectal space (transsphincteric fistula).[5]

The cause of perianal fistulas in Crohn disease may be a fistula arising from inflamed or infected anal glands, and/or penetration of fissures or ulcers in the rectum or anal canal.[8–10]

DIAGNOSIS: ACCURACY AND APPLICATION OF MR IMAGING

The use of MR imaging in the evaluation of perianal fistulas has been reported in many studies,[11–13] showing it to be the preferred technique for preoperative evaluation of perianal fistulas and improved patient outcome.[4] MR imaging has a

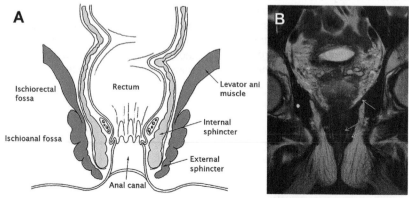

Fig. 2. Drawing (*A*) and T2-weighted image (*B*) show the normal anatomy of the perianal region in the coronal plane. *Arrows* indicate internal and external sphincter.

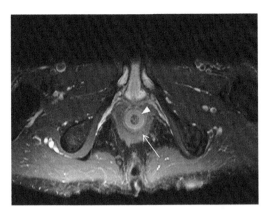

Fig. 3. Normal anatomy of the anal sphincter complex on axial T1-weighted image after administration of gadolinium. Note the high degree of enhancement of the internal sphincter (*arrowheads*) compared with the intermediate signal intensity of the external sphincter (*arrows*).

high sensitivity and specificity in the detection of primary and secondary tracks, abscesses, and internal openings.

Endoscopic ultrasound can be equivalent to MR imaging in complementing examination under anesthesia.[14] In clinical practice, MR imaging is used more frequently than endoscopic ultrasound. Endoscopic ultrasound is operator-dependent, and in patients with severe proctitis or anal strictures, its tolerability is suboptimal. Furthermore, the limited field of view is a considerable inconvenience, precluding the use of endoscopic ultrasound to assess suprasphincteric and extrasphincteric tracks or secondary extensions.[4]

Several studies have reported that preoperative pelvic MR imaging findings change surgical management in 10% to 15% of patients,[14–16] or reveal important additional information in 21% of patients, particularly those with Crohn disease.[13]

In a larger study of patients with a recurrent anal fistula, the postoperative recurrence rate was as low as 16% when surgeons always acted based on the MR imaging findings. The rate of recurrence was 30% when surgeons occasionally acted based on MR imaging results, and 57% when MR imaging results were ignored.[4,17]

Currently, MR imaging is also a reliable technique to assess the outcome of medical therapy using the anti-TNF agent infliximab in patients with Crohn disease with fistula-in-ano occurring during the first year of follow-up (**Fig. 4**).[18] This result was confirmed by 3 similar studies[19–21] and also by another study using endoscopic ultrasound.[22]

However, in the long-term follow-up, the improvements observed at MR imaging correlate with the clinical and endoscopic response to infliximab in only half of the patients.[23]

MR IMAGING PROTOCOL/TECHNIQUE

Various MR imaging techniques have been described.[4,24]

Imaging Coils

Two types of coils can be used: the endoanal and the external phased array coils. Use of endoanal coils was initially proposed to improve MR imaging evaluation of perianal fistulas, but these coils are poorly tolerated in symptomatic patients.[4,25]

Advantages of the external phased array coil include the larger field of view, which prevents fistula extensions from being overlooked, especially in patients with Crohn disease, and the wide availability of these coils. Furthermore, MR imaging with phased array surface coils requires no patient preparation and is well tolerated.

Imaging Sequences

On T2-weighted MR sequences, active fistulas and abscesses are hyperintense.[2]

T1-weighted contrast-enhanced fat-suppressed MR imaging sequences are used to further improve the contrast of pelvic MR imaging and to distinguish inflamed tissue from normal perineal tissues.[25,26] Furthermore, images with fat suppression better illustrate the activity of the fistulas.[18]

A gadolinium-enhanced T1-weighted sequence is helpful in differentiating between fluid and granulation tissue, which is important in abscesses. Pus has high signal intensity on T2-weighted images, and thus cannot be reliably distinguished from edema and inflammation. The use of dynamic contrast-enhanced MR imaging for determining the degree of activity in perianal Crohn disease might be helpful in selecting a subpopulation of patients with perianal Crohn disease who should be monitored more closely for development of more extensive disease.[27]

Another recent development is the introduction of 3.0-Tesla (T) imaging. 3.0-T imaging further improves spatial resolution and secondary diagnostic accuracy.[28] The finer detail helps in detecting and characterizing even smaller fistula tracks. However, comparative studies with 1.5-T or 3.0-T have not been reported.

Use of diffusion-weighted sequences for evaluating perianal fistulas has been reported.[29] Because inflammatory tissues usually have high signal intensity at diffusion-weighted imaging, this technique is used as an adjunct to T2-weighted imaging for diagnosing anal fistulas.

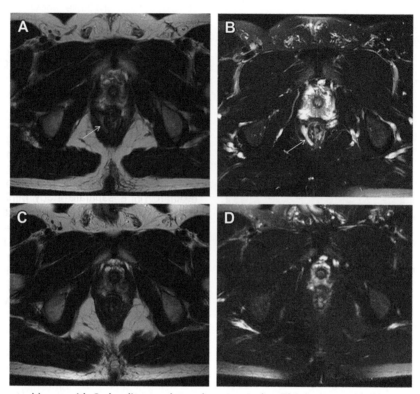

Fig. 4. A 37-year-old man with Crohn disease who underwent a subtotal colectomy with ileorectal anastomosis. T2-weighted MR images without (*A*) and with (*B*) fat suppression before treatment show an intersphincteric fistula at the right side (*arrows*). (*C, D*) Short-term MR imaging follow-up (10 weeks) after infliximab treatment (5 mg/kg) shows disappearance of the fistula.

Imaging Planes

Another important advantage of MR imaging is the multiplanar assessment. However, imaging planes must be correctly aligned to the anal canal. Therefore, a sequence in the sagittal plane is first performed. The transverse and coronal sequences must be aligned with the anal canal at the sagittal sequence, oriented perpendicularly (transverse) and parallel (sagittal) to the long axis of the anal canal.[4]

The specific protocol and sequence parameters applied at the authors' institution are provided in detail in the first table: sagittal fat-suppressed T2-weighted turbo spin echo (TSE), axial fat-suppressed T2-weighted TSE, axial oblique T2-weighted TSE (short axis), coronal oblique T2-weighted TSE (long axis), and axial oblique and coronal oblique fat-suppressed T1-weighted TSE with gadolinium (**Table 1**).

CLASSIFICATION

Fistulas may be classified according to the course of the fistula from the anal canal to the skin and its relationships to the internal and external sphincters.

In 1976, Parks and colleagues[30] proposed an anatomic precise classification system for perianal fistulas that uses the external sphincter as a central point of reference. This classification was developed primarily for surgical treatment and is therefore especially important for patients treated surgically.

Five types of perianal fistulas were described: intersphincteric, transsphincteric, suprasphincteric, extrasphincteric, and superficial.

1. Intersphincteric fistulas course from the internal opening in the anal canal through the internal sphincter and the intersphincteric plane to the perianal skin. The fistula is entirely confined by the external sphincter; the ischiorectal and ischioanal fossae are unaffected (**Fig. 5**).
2. Instead of tracking down the intersphincteric plane to the skin, the transsphincteric fistula perforates through both layers of the sphincter complex into the ischiorectal and ischioanal fossae (**Fig. 6**).
3. Less frequent is a suprasphincteric fistula, wherein the tract passes upward in the intersphincteric plane over the top of the puborectal muscle and then descends through the levator plate to the ischioanal fossa and finally to the skin (**Fig. 7**).

Table 1
MR imaging protocol

Scan Parameters	Scan Name					
	T2_TSE_sagittal_FS	T2_TSE_axial_FS	T2_TSE_axial oblique	T2_TSE_coronal oblique	T1_TSE_axial oblique_FS	T1_TSE_coronal oblique_FS
Sequence type	Turbo spin echo (TSE)	Turbo spin echo (TSE)	Turbo spin echo (TSE)	Turbo spin echo (TSE)	Turbo spin echo (TSE)	Turbo spin echo (TSE)
Orientation	Sagittal	Axial	Axial oblique	Coronal oblique	Axial oblique	Coronal oblique
Number of slices	20	30	20	20	26	20
Slice thickness (mm)	4	6	6	6	4	4
Slice gap (mm)	0.8	1.2	1.26	1.26	0	0
Field of View (mm)	259 × 360	230 × 320	230 × 320	270 × 320	309 × 380	380 × 380
TR (ms)	8870	6960	8870	8780	730	580
TE (ms)	134	134	134	134	11	11
Number of averages	3	4	3	2	3	3
Fat suppression	Yes	Yes	No	No	Yes	Yes
Matrix	368 × 512	368 × 512	368 × 512	432 × 512	416 × 512	512 × 512
Pixel resolution (mm)	0.7 × 0.7 × 4.0	0.6 × 0.6 × 6.0	0.6 × 0.6 × 6.0	0.6 × 0.6 × 6.0	0.7 × 0.7 × 4.0	0.7 × 0.7 × 4.0
Acquisition time (min:s)	1:39	3:16	1:30	1:38	5:48	5:39
Extra information			Orientation axial to anal canal	Orientation coronal to anal canal	Acquired twice, once before and once after contrast administration, axial to anal canal	After contrast administration, coronal to anal canal
Less commonly mentioned, but can be added if desired						
Parallel imaging	GRAPPA, factor 2	GRAPPA, factor 2	GRAPPA, factor 2	GRAPPA, factor 2	GRAPPA, factor 2	GRAPPA, factor 2
Bandwidth (Hz/Px)	305	305	305	305	195	195
Turbo factor	61	61	61	61	3	3

Parameters were established with the Aera 1.5 Tesla system (Siemens, Erlangen, Germany).
Abbreviations: FS, fat suppression; GRAPPA, Generalized Autocalibrating Partially Parallel Acquisitions; Hz, hertz; Px, pixel; T1, T1-weighted; T2, T2-weighted; TSE, turbo spin echo.

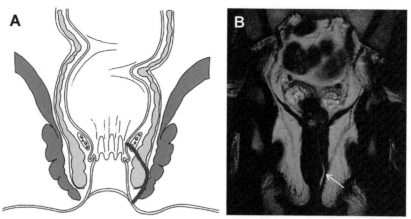

Fig. 5. Drawing (*A*) and T2-weighted image (*B*) in the coronal plane show a left intersphincteric fistula (*A; red line, B; arrow*) extending from the anal canal to the skin, crossing through the intersphincteric space.

4. Relatively rare are extrasphincteric fistulas in which the tract passes from the rectal mucosa through the ischioanal fossa and levator muscles to the skin. This type of fistula lies outside the anal sphincter complex, and the anal canal is not involved (**Fig. 8**).
5. Superficial fistulas were not included in the original publication by Parks and colleagues,[30] but have been added to the classification. These fistulas do not involve the anal sphincter complex, and MR imaging is not needed routinely.

MR GRADING OF PERIANAL FISTULAS

Through adding MR imaging findings, the St James's University Hospital classification became

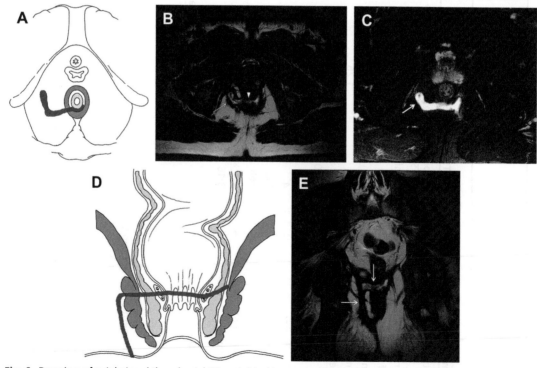

Fig. 6. Drawing of axial view (*A*) and axial T2-weighted images without (*B*) and with (*C*) fat suppression show a right transsphincteric fistula (*A; red line*) crossing both layers of the sphincter complex, complicated by an abscess (*B, C; arrows*) in the right ischiorectal fossa, with an internal opening at the 6 o'clock position (*B; arrowheads*). Drawing of coronal view (*D*) and coronal T2-weighted image without fat suppression (*E*) show the craniocaudal extension of the fistula in the right ischiorectal fossa (*D; red line, E; arrows*).

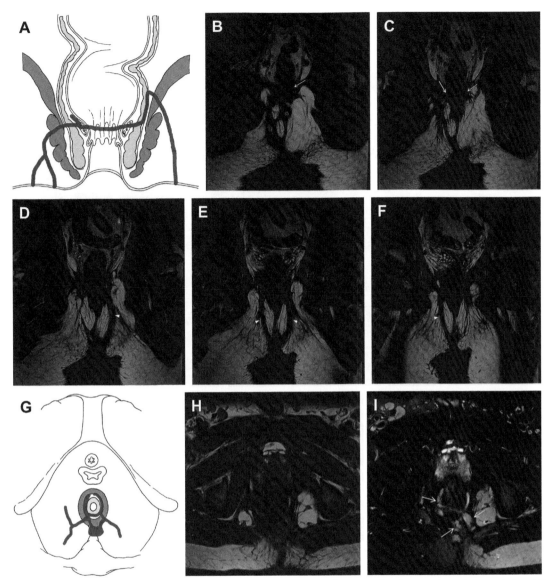

Fig. 7. A 35-year-old man with Crohn disease and a complex suprasphincteric fistula. Drawing of coronal view (*A*) and coronal (*B–F*) T1-weighted image after administration of gadolinium show upward fistula extensions through the intersphincteric space, over the top of the levator ani muscle (*A; red line, B* and *C; arrows*). The fistulas then descend through the ischiorectal fossa at both sides to reach the skin (*D–F; arrowheads*). Drawing in axial view (*G*) and axial T2-weighted images without (*H*) and with (*I*) fat suppression show the extensive supralevator horseshoe ramifications (*G; red line, H* and *I; arrows*).

a morphologic assessment of the location of anal fistulas to the sphincter complex to guide the surgical management.[5]

The score ranges from 1 to 5 and indicates the primary fistulous track and the secondary ramifications and associated abscesses.

Grade 1: Single Intersphincteric Fistula

A single intersphincteric fistula extends from the skin to the anal canal in the plane between the sphincters. There is no ramification of the fistula within the sphincter complex, and the ischioanal and ischiorectal fossae are unaffected at MR imaging.

Grade 2: Single or Multibranched Intersphincteric Fistula with Abscess

Intersphincteric fistulas with an abscess or secondary track are confined within the sphincter (horseshoe fistula or abscess).

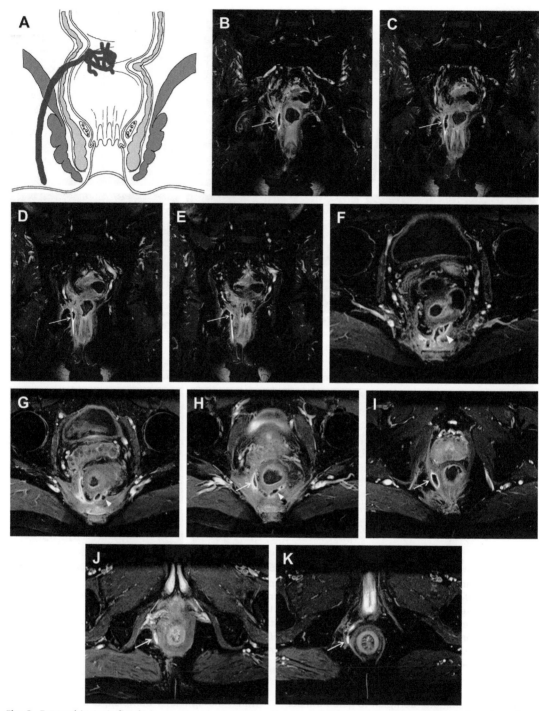

Fig. 8. Extrasphincteric fistula in a patient with known diverticulitis of the sigmoid (*A; red line*). Drawing of coronal view (*A*) and coronal (*B–E*) and axial (*F–K*) T1-weighted images after administration of gadolinium show inflammatory changes surrounding the rectum (supralevator disease) (*F–H; arrowheads*) and the right translevator fistula crossing the ischiorectal fossa, outside the sphincter complex (*B–E, H–K; arrows*).

Grade 3: Unbranched Transsphincteric Fistula

Unbranched transsphincteric fistulas extend through both layers of the sphincter complex with extensions in the ischioanal or ischiorectal fossa.

Grade 4: Transsphincteric Fistula with Abscess or Secondary Track Within the Ischiorectal or Ischioanal Fossa

A transsphincteric fistula can be complicated by sepsis in the ischiorectal or ischioanal fossa.

Grade 5: Translevatoric or Supralevatoric Fistula

In rare cases, fistulas extend above the levator ani muscle. Suprasphincteric fistulas extend upward in the intersphincteric plane and over the top of the levator ani; extrasphincteric fistulas are extensions of primary pelvic disease down through the levator plate.

This MR imaging classification is significantly associated with patient outcome ($P<.001$). MR imaging grades 1 and 2 were associated with a satisfactory outcome (no further surgery needed), whereas grades 3 through 5 were associated with unsatisfactory outcome (further surgery needed).[5]

To provide a more accurate evaluation of disease activity, the Leuven MR imaging–based activity score was developed to evaluate the activity of anal fistulas of patients with Crohn disease during medical treatment (**Fig. 9**).[18] This score correlates with clinical disease activity and response to medical therapy. Both anatomic parameters and parameters reflecting active inflammation are evaluated in the MR imaging score. Anatomic criteria are based on the Parks classification. The location of the primary track (intersphincteric, transsphincteric, or extrasphincteric) and the extension (infralevatoric or supralevatoric), and the complexity of the track (single, single-branched, or multiple) are described.

Criteria of fistula activity are T2 hyperintense appearance of the fistula track, presence of hyperintense cavities, and thickening of the rectal wall (**Table 2**). The MR imaging score was reliable in assessing the fistula tracks, with a good interobserver concordance ($P<.001$).[18]

Despite the closure of draining external orifices after infliximab therapy, fistula tracks persist with varying degrees of residual inflammation, which may cause recurrent fistulas and pelvic abscesses. More specifically, the inflammatory components of the score improve more consistently than the anatomic criteria, indicating that fistula tracks can persist while inflammation is subsiding.[18]

Gadolinium-enhanced T1-weighted images are not used in the Leuven MR imaging–based score.[18] Some authors, however, have found that fistulas are more conspicuous on these images than on T2-weighted images.[31,32] Hyperintensity

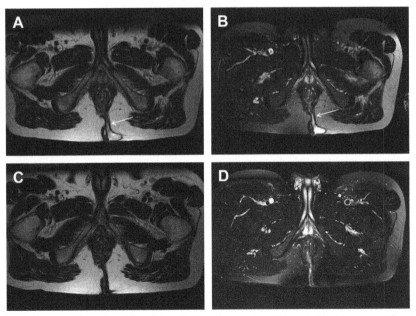

Fig. 9. A 49-year-old man with perianal fistulizing Crohn disease. Axial T2-weighted images without (A) and with (B) fat suppression before treatment show an active transsphincteric fistula (arrows): severe T2 hyperintensity of the fistula track. MR imaging score: 19/22. After treatment, the fistula track is still present but is rather inactive, as evident by the hypointensity on the T2-weighted images (C, D). MR imaging score: 11/22.

Table 2
MR imaging–based score for severity of perianal Crohn disease

Number of fistula tracks	
None	0
Single, unbranched	1
Single, branched	2
Multiple	3
Location	
Extrasphincteric or intersphincteric	1
Transsphincteric	2
Suprasphincteric	3
Extension	
Infralevatoric	1
Supralevatoric	2
Hyperintensity on T2-weighted images	
Absent	0
Mild	4
Pronounced	8
Collections (cavities >3 mm diameter)	
Absent	0
Present	4
Rectal wall involvement	
Normal	0
Thickened	2

Data from Van Assche G, Vanbeckevoort D, Bielen D, et al. Magnetic resonance imaging of the effects of infliximab on perianal fistulizing Crohn disease. Am J Gastroenterol 2003;98(2):332–9.

on T1 can be seen from increased tissue perfusion and vascular permeability.[33] As local vascularization and permeability increase with the severity of inflammatory disease, the postcontrast enhancement of inflammatory tissue reflects the degree of inflammatory activity of the tissue.[34,35]

The Leuven MR imaging–based score of disease severity can be used to evaluate response to treatment with infliximab remission induction therapy. One study noted a clinical response in 44% of patients, but a relapse was observed in 57% of these patients.[21] In all 4 relapsing patients, MR imaging scores were indicative of persistence of active perianal fistulizing disease. The inclusion of contrast enhancement or tissue infiltration does not add value to the MR imaging–based score.[21]

SUMMARY

Imaging now plays an important role in the surgical and nonsurgical evaluation of anal fistulas. High-resolution MR imaging is currently the preferred technique, allowing precise assessment of the relationship between the fistula track and the pelvic floor structures, and identification of secondary fistulas or abscesses.

The St James's University Hospital MR imaging classification is developed to give the exact location and characteristics of the fistula track to guide surgeons in their surgical approach.

With the development in medical therapy, clinicians now want to know the actual status or activity of the fistula disease. It guides their decisions whether to start or continue medical treatment, or whether surgical intervention is warranted.

The Leuven MR imaging–based activity score was specifically developed to evaluate the activity of anal fistulas, especially in patients with Crohn disease. This score correlates well with clinical disease activity and the response to medical treatment.

ACKNOWLEDGMENTS

All drawings used in this article were created by Patricia Poels.

REFERENCES

1. Sainio P. Fistula-in-ano in a defined population. Incidence and epidemiological aspects. Ann Chir Gynaecol 1984;73:219–24.
2. Ziech M, Felt-Bersma R, Stoker J. Imaging of perianal fistulas. Clin Gastroenterol Hepatol 2009;7:1037–45.
3. Eisenhammer S. A new approach to the anorectal fistulous abscess based on the high intermuscular lesion. Surg Gynecol Obstet 1958;106(5):595–9.
4. de Miguel Criado J, del Salto LG, Rivas PF, et al. MR imaging of perianal fistulas: spectrum of imaging features. Radiographics 2012;32:175–94.
5. Morris J, Spencer JA, Ambrose NS. MR imaging classification of perianal fistulas and its implications for patient management. Radiographics 2000;20:623–35.
6. deSouza NM, Puni R, Kmiot WA, et al. MRI of the anal sphincter. J Comput Assist Tomogr 1995;19:745–51.
7. Schaefer O, Oeksuez MO, Lohrmann C, et al. Differentiation of anal sphincters with high-resolution magnetic resonance imaging using contrast-enhanced fast low-angle shot 3-dimensional sequences. J Comput Assist Tomogr 2004;28:174–9.
8. Parks AG. Pathogenesis and treatment of fistula-in-ano. Br Med J 1961;1:463–9.
9. Sandborn WJ, Fazio VW, Feagan BG, et al. AGA technical review on perianal Crohn's disease. Gastroenterology 2003;125(5):1508–30.

10. Hughes LE. Surgical pathology and management of anorectal Crohn's disease. J R Soc Med 1978;71(9): 644–51.

11. Hussain SM, Stoker J, Schouten WR, et al. Fistula in ano: endoanal sonography versus endoanal MR imaging in classification. Radiology 1996;200(2): 475–81.

12. deSouza NM, Gilderdale DJ, Coutts GA, et al. MRI of fistula-in-ano: a comparison of endoanal coil with external phased array coil techniques. J Comput Assist Tomogr 1998;22(3):357–63.

13. Beets-Tan RG, Beets GL, van der Hoop AG, et al. Preoperative MR imaging of anal fistulas: does it really help the surgeon? Radiology 2001;218:75–84.

14. Schwartz DA, Wiersema MJ, Dudiak KM, et al. A comparison of endoscopic ultrasound, magnetic resonance imaging, and exam under anesthesia for evaluation of Crohn's perianal fistulas. Gastroenterology 2001;121:1064–72.

15. deSouza NM, Hall AS, Puni R, et al. High resolution magnetic resonance imaging of the anal sphincter using a dedicated endoanal coil. Comparison of magnetic resonance imaging with surgical findings. Dis Colon Rectum 1996;39:926–34.

16. Spencer JA, Chapple K, Wilson D, et al. Outcome after surgery for perianal fistula: predictive value of MR imaging. Am J Roentgenol 1998;171:403–6.

17. Buchanan G, Halligan S, Williams A, et al. Effect of MRI on clinical outcome of recurrent fistula-in-ano. Lancet 2002;360(9346):1661–2.

18. Van Assche G, Vanbeckevoort D, Bielen D, et al. Magnetic resonance imaging of the effects of infliximab on perianal fistulizing Crohn's disease. Am J Gastroenterol 2003;98:332–9.

19. Bell SJ, Halligan S, Windsor AC, et al. Response of fistulating Crohn's disease to infliximab treatment assessed by magnetic resonance imaging. Aliment Pharmacol Ther 2003;17(3):387–93.

20. Ng SC, Plamondon S, Gupta A, et al. Prospective evaluation of anti-tumor necrosis factor therapy guided by magnetic resonance imaging for Crohn's perianal fistulas. Am J Gastroenterol 2009;104: 2973–86.

21. Horsthuis K, Ziech ML, Bipat S, et al. Evaluation of an MRI-based score of disease activity in perianal fistulizing Crohn's disease. Clin Imaging 2011;35:360–5.

22. Van Bodegraven AA, Sloots CE, Felt-Bersma RJ, et al. Endosonographic evidence of persistence of Crohn's disease-associated fistulas after infliximab treatment, irrespective of clinical response. Dis Colon Rectum 2002;45(1):39–45.

23. Karmiris K, Bielen D, Vanbeckevoort D, et al. Long-term monitoring of infliximab therapy for perianal fistulizing Crohn's disease by using magnetic resonance imaging. Clin Gastroenterol Hepatol 2011; 9(2):130–6.

24. Stoker J, Rociu E, Zwamborn AW, et al. Endoluminal MR imaging of the rectum and anus: technique, applications, and pitfalls. Radiographics 1999;19: 383–98.

25. Halligan S, Bartram CI. MR imaging of fistula in ano: are endoanal coils the gold standard? Am J Roentgenol 1998;171(2):407–12.

26. Halligan S, Stoker J. Imaging of fistula-in-ano. Radiology 2006;239(1):18–33.

27. Horsthuis K, Lavini C, Bipat S, et al. Perianal Crohn disease: evaluation of dynamic contrast-enhanced MR imaging as an indicator of disease activity. Radiology 2009;251(2):380–7.

28. Chang KJ, Kamel IR, Macura KJ, et al. 3.0 T MR imaging of the abdomen: comparison with 1.5 T. Radiographics 2008;28(7):1983–98.

29. Hori M, Oto A, Orrin S, et al. Diffusion-weighted MRI: a new tool for the diagnosis of fistula in ano. J Magn Reson Imaging 2009;30(5):1021–6.

30. Parks AG, Gordon PH, Hardcastle JD. A classification of fistula-in-ano. Br J Surg 1976;63:1–12.

31. Semelka RC, Hricak H, Kim B, et al. Pelvic fistulas: appearances on MR images. Abdom Imaging 1997;22:91–5.

32. Schmidt S, Chevallier P, Bessoud B, et al. Diagnostic performance of MRI for detection of intestinal fistulas in patients with complicated inflammatory bowel conditions. Eur Radiol 2007;17:2957–63.

33. Weinmann HJ, Brasch RC, Press WR, et al. Characteristics of gadolinium-DPTA complex: a potential NMR contrast agent. Am J Roentgenol 1984;142: 619–24.

34. Brahme F, Lindstrom C. A comparative radiographic and pathological study of intestinal vasoarchitecture in Crohn's disease and in ulcerative colitis. Gut 1970;11:928–40.

35. Van Dijke CF, Peterfy CG, Brasch RC, et al. MR imaging of the arthritic rabbit knee joint using albumin-(Gd-DPTA)30 with correlation to histopathology. Magn Reson Imaging 1999;17:237–45.

Index

Note: Page numbers of article titles are in **boldface** type.

A

Adenocarcinomas, of small bowel, MR enteroclysis of, 55–56, 57
Adenoma(s), benign villous, 97
   of small bowel, MR enteroclysis in, 54
Anal canal, normal anatomy of, 113–114, 115
Anal cancer, and rectal cancer, MR imaging of, **85–112**
   involving vagina and urethra, 109, 110
   MR imaging of, 107–111
      N and M staging of, 109–111
      T staging in, 107–109
   of anal canal at pelvic floor, 109, 110, 111
   squamous cell cancer above anal canal, 107, 109
Anti-peristaltics, for MR enterography, 5

B

Bowel, diffusion-weighted imaging of, 8–9
   MR imaging of, techniques of, **1–11**
   peristalsis of, cine imaging to assess, 9
   small, benign tumors of, 53–55
      lipomas of, T1-weighted imaging in, 55
      malignant tumors of, 55–62
      MR imaging of, in Crohn disease, **13–22**
         techniques for, 13–14
      noninflammatory conditions of, **51–65**
         image interpretation in, 53
         MR enteroclysis in, 53
         MR enterography in, 52–53
         MR imaging in, 51
            contrast agents for, 52
            technical considerations in, 52–53
            reduction of peristalsis in, 53
      wall of, in Crohn disease, MR imaging findings in, 39–40, 41, 42
         thickening of, 43
Bowel disease, inflammatory. See *Inflammatory bowel disease*.

C

Celiac disease, MR enterography in, 60–62
   MR imaging in, 52
Chemical shift imaging, 9
Cine imaging, to assess bowel peristalsis, 9
Colon, luminal inflammation of, in Crohn disease, 24–25
   normal anatomy of, 68

Colonography, 1
   MR. See *MR colonography*.
Colorectal cancer, complicating inflammatory bowel disease, MR colonography and, 28–29
   development from colorectal polyps, 69
   differential diagnosis of, using MR colonography, 70
   diverticulitis mimicking, 78
   incidence of, 67
   MR colonography for screening and diagnosis of, **67–83**
   pathology of, 68–69
   screening tools for, 67
   survival rate for, 67
Contrast, colonic, for MR enterography, 4
   intravenous, for MR enterography, 5–6
   small bowel, for MR enterography, 2–4
Crohn disease, abnormal peristalsis in, MR motility imaging of, 40–41
   active inflammatory, 15, 19
      and fibrostenosing, differentiation of, 16–19, 20
   classification of, 14
   clinical prsentation of, 36
   colonic luminal inflammation in, 24–25
   complications of, 43
   diagnosis of, 23, 36
   enteroenteric fistula in, 43
   fibrostenosing, 15–16
      and active inflammatory, differentiation of, 16–19, 20
   imaging findings in, 15–19
   imaging techniques used in, 23–24
   inflammation of mesentery in, comb sign in, 41–42
   management of, 36
   mesenteric lymphadenopathy in, 42–43
   mixed fibrostenosing, and active inflammatory, 19, 20
   MR enterography in, 15–19, 20
   MR imaging of small bowel in, **13–22**
      techniques for, 13–14
   new MR imaging modalities for, **35–50**
   pathology of, 35
   penetrating, 16, 17, 18
   perianal, severity of, MR imaging-based score for, 122
   perianal disease in, 43–45
   perianal fistulizing, 121
   severe rectal inflammation secondary to, 26–27, 28
   small bowel in, MR imaging findings in, 39–45

mri.theclinics.com

Moving?

Make sure your subscription moves with you!

To notify us of your new address, find your **Clinics Account Number** (located on your mailing label above your name), and contact customer service at:

Email: journalscustomerservice-usa@elsevier.com

800-654-2452 (subscribers in the U.S. & Canada)
314-447-8871 (subscribers outside of the U.S. & Canada)

Fax number: 314-447-8029

Elsevier Health Sciences Division
Subscription Customer Service
3251 Riverport Lane
Maryland Heights, MO 63043

Printed and bound by CPI Group (UK) Ltd, Croydon, CR0 4YY

03/10/2024

01040370-0003